Dr. Vinod Verma

Yog

A Natural Way of Being

A nine-week, easy-to-do programme for initiation into adopting yoga as a way of life

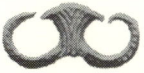

Gayatri Books International

The information provided in this book is not intended to replace the services of a physician. The suggestions for a healthy way of living with yoga provided in this book are for the purpose of self-help and education. The author and the publisher are in no way responsible for any medical claims regarding the material presented in this book. For using methods and remedies provided in this book at commercial level requires the prior permission from the author. For more information, write to the author directly at ayurvedavv@yahoo.com

Translation rights are with the author. The book is already published in German, French, English, Slovenian, Italian and Hindi. Write to the author directly at ayurvedavv@yahoo.com or ayurvedavv@gmail.com for translation rights.

Visit Dr. Vinod Verma at www.ayurvedavv.com and www.drvinodverma.com to find out about her seminars, lectures and consultations, etc. Information is also provided at the back pages of the book.

Consultant: Mohit Joshi
Design and photographs by the author

ISBN: 978-1495484209

Yoga

A Natural Way of Being

- ❖ With a simple nine-week-plan, let your-self be initiated into yoga as your way of life.
- ❖ Learn to be as spontaneous and natural as a child.
- ❖ Learn the right way to stand, walk, think and breathe through this yoga plan.
- ❖ Correct your posture and cure your aches and pains through simple yogic exercises.
- ❖ Enhance your body flexibility and mental capabilities.

Dedicated

To My Late Father

Shree Om Prakash from whom I learnt the
first yogasanas

A Word for the Present Edition

This book was written in 1987 when I was living in Germany and France. It is a basic book to initiate people into making yoga as a way of life. During the past 27 years, this book has been published in six different languages and several editions in each language. I still continue to get reader's mail from all over the world including my own country.

A revised International edition was published in 2006. In these 27 years, I have written and published 23 more books on various aspects of yoga and Ayurveda as well as on women and companionship. The basic value of this book remains, as it was several decades ago—to initiate the beginners into a yogic way of life for health and harmony.

The world over, more and more young people are getting aware that the solution to good health and peaceful life lies in taking responsibility for oneself and not depending on the doctors to 'mend the body machine' in case of ailments. Besides that, the fundamental wisdom of yoga teaches us the basic values of life which are missing in the education imparted at home these days. We are going through times when everybody says: 'I do not have time'. Parents do not have time for children and children do not have time for parents. When awareness triggers at certain age, young people look for some guidance and this kind of a short and simple book on basic wisdom of life can help them as a guide.

I am grateful to my readers in various countries for their enthusiasm for this book.

Vinod Verma
www.ayurvedavv.com ayurvedavv@yahoo.com
ayurvedavv@yahoo.com
January 2014

Yoga: A Natural Way of Being

Foreword

Dr. Vinod Verma's 'Yoga for Integral Health' has already become a mini-classic both in Europe and India. In this 9-week, easy to manage yoga course, she has managed to condense, with enviable lucidity and simplicity, wisdom, knowledge, information and technique of centuries, if not millennia.

Pertinently she draws attention to the fundamental premise of the worldview on which a system of comprehending the body-mind-soul relationship is grounded. No holistic system of medicine could have emerged from an opposite worldview of binary opposites, mind-body, subject-object, dualities. Thus, before embarking upon the journey of the 9-week easy-to-manage yoga course, any serious discerning reader has to be acquainted with the deeper layers of the sources of thought and speculation which facilitated the organic growth of a highly integrated system of medicine and understanding of the body.

Dr. Vinod Verma commences her book thoughtfully with two introductory chapters, which elucidate the worldview - history and philosophic background. This was altogether necessary in a situation that the enigmatic word 'yoga' has been of late used and much abused out of context at the most superficial levels. Commodification of 'concepts' denoting 'wholeness' for ready consumption of a fractured world and out of joint mind and body is not uncommon. This is another indicator of the spell and attraction of the reductionist model in our contemporary world. Dr. Verma with the assistance of simple anecdotes and personal narrations succeeds in dispelling some of these notions. Her first and last plea is for 'integration' and wholeness. The body system she dwells upon is an intrinsic part of that totality and cannot and must not be isolated. Yoga thus is neither acrobatics nor gymnastics; it is a system of realising the body, mind and consciousness.

Her pointed reference to the attitude to the 'body' and the comprehension of the body and its parts is of utmost importance. The Sanskrit word sharira, neither in its connotative nor denotive meanings, refers to the skeletal frame and the muscular and other systems, while this understanding is subsumed in the word sharira. In the Indian tradition, the body has been viewed as an 'abode' or instrument of the 'soul' (i.e., atman). However, this abode or temple of the divine, i.e. body, is subject to decay and death, to be enshrined again and again in other bodies. There are many cognates of the one word sharira, such as deha, tanu kshetra, anga, etc. Each of these emphasises that at the conceptual level the body (sharira) is the house of the divine, atman. It is not sentient by itself. Also, that as structure it is organic, made up of the appropriate but not fixed confluence of the five primal elements, panchabhuta, viz., space, air, fire, water and earth. The harmonious balance of the elements within the body is the quintessence of physical, emotional and psychical health. Sharira thus is the repository of everything, specially mind, speech, vital force (prana). Sharira in its very nature is of course transient and ephemeral. The Brihadaranyaka Upanishad draws attention to the return of the body to the primal elements. 'The speech of the dead returns to the fire, his breath returns to air, his eyes to the sun, his mind to the moon, his ears to the directions of space and his body to earth'. Another Upanishad, namely, the Taittiriya, speaks of the inter-dependence of the body (sharira) and soul (atman) (prana). 'The body rests in prana and the prana is seated in the body'.

The perception cited above could be elaborated upon a hundred-fold. In the context of Dr. Vinod Verma's book it is well to be conscious of this background and attitude. The body then is not an instrument of attraction, temptation; it is indeed a 'sacred' entity for comprehending the inner and outer self. To maintain the instrument in perfect balance and harmony is an essential pre-requisite of the totality of life. 'Yoga' thus is not an alternate to modern day 'beauty parlours'! Dr. Verma's book urges the reader to make this paradigmical shift before commencing on the 9-week logically structured course.

At the level of information, techniques of awareness and motor movements of the different parts of the body (anga) and pratiyanga, she proceeds cautiously but with precision. As a dancer and student of the Natyasastra, as also Sangitaratnakara, for me the chapters were of great interest. The texts of music and dance devote considerable attention to understanding the body, its parts and centres of motor movements and breath regulation and speech centres. Dr. Verma's brief, pithy explanations and guidance will no doubt guide the learner effectively, but these chapters contain the kernel of further inter-disciplinary work which needs to be done to explicate the connections between and amongst the diverse domains of knowledge and disciplines. Dr. Verma has touched upon the metaphysical dimensions. Equally pertinent are the dimensions of the close and integral relationship between systems of 'yoga' and the arts of India. This is a level of the integration of the body, mind and consciousness in concepts of on all creativity in the Indian tradition.

I have no doubt that the re-publication of the revised international edition of the book will be received with as much enthusiasm and it will no doubt benefit all those who wish to aspire for an integrated life style.

Kapila Vatsyayan
New Delhi
April 28, 2004

11

Yoga: A Natural Way of Being

Preface

The word 'yoga' is one of the most exploited words of our time. During the past twenty-five years, it has been made to mean and represent different ideas, the most frequent of them being a kind of physical exercise with a mystical meaning. Sometimes, it is also associated with acrobatics. Professor Jean Varenne has put my point in apt words: 'Yoga—a with-it word perpetually catching the eye from posters, from covers of garishly printed magazines, and needless to say, from publishers' catalogs. ... "I do yoga every Friday afternoon, I find it relaxes me"; someone else "does yoga" to help his bad back; another "to keep a clear head at work". Almost everywhere you find flourishing "schools of yoga" that teach a sort of Swedish drill interspersed with pauses for breathing: ... The teacher twists himself into bizarre contortions, ... the clients themselves venture no further than simply sitting cross-legged on the floor; and even that they find uncomfortable and difficult to keep for very long.[1]

People who sincerely wish to know what yoga is and what is the purpose of various yogic practices have a genuine difficulty in finding an appropriate teacher and book. Most of the existing books on yogic practices turn 'yoga' into mere slowed down gymnastics. There are other books on the practice of yoga which make the exposition of the discipline in a very traditional Hindu way which many people find difficult to subscribe to. They face physical difficulties in learning yogic postures on the one hand and to comprehend the philosophical aspects of the discipline on the other hand.

Being a medical scientist and at the same time brought up with the yogic tradition, I found myself in a position to write a

---

[1] *Jean Varenne,* Yoga and the Hindu Tradition, *page vii, 1976, TheUniversity of Chicago Press, Chicago*

simple book on the subject where first of all the metaphysical meaning of the discipline is made clear to show that this practice leads one to the path of self-realisation and consciousness.

Secondly, the yogic practices are taught progressively with many preparatory physical and mental exercises. The traditional postures and concentration practices are aspired to after body and mind have acquired a pre-requisite for them. Most of my adult life, I have stayed in Europe and also partly in the United States. My practical experience in giving yoga courses to the people there has helped me to see the physical and mental difficulties in the path of the yoga aspirant.

Although the Yoga Sutras or aphorisms of the philosopher and the teacher Patanjali (estimated date 500 B.C.) are the first written text which made yoga a philosophical discipline, the yogic practices existed in India as early as 3,000 B.C. This antiquity is ascertained from the seals and sculptures of the Indus Valley civilization showing several yogic postures. I feel that before taking up any aspect of this ancient discipline which has come to us from time immemorial, it is very important to understand it. To make comprehension easier, it is necessary to present the ideas in a lucid way and to put them in their historical perspective. After comprehension, comes the practical aspect. My emphasis in this direction is on a very gradual progression. Yoga being a very ancient practice, yogasanas (yoga postures) were adapted according to the lifestyle of the earlier people. Human beings were required to work more with their bodies during those days. Life was more restful on our planet earth. Although the people did not have so many of the material luxuries of today, they were blessed with a greater flexibility of mind and body. During the last few centuries, we have lost this and we have become stiffer physically as well as mentally. Thus, it is difficult to learn the yogic practices by beginning with their traditional form as we no more have the pre-requisite of a relaxed mind and the flexibility of body. We have to prepare ourselves physically and mentally before taking the path of yoga.

14

To elucidate my above statement, I would compare learning of yogic practices to learning a new language. Someone who knows English before beginning to learn French, has not only the advantage of knowing Latin alphabet beforehand but also has a facility due to the common origin of these two languages. Thus, the learning of this new language starts from a certain pre-supposed level. However, if this person wants to learn Chinese, he or she will have to start from the very beginning.

A course of yogic practices offered in this book is very fundamental and is basically designed for the maintenance of good physical and mental health. No spiritual path is possible without the physical well-being. The body[2] is holy because it houses the soul, which according to the yoga tradition is a part of the Absolute.

The hectic life in technologically advanced countries and in all big cities of the world has made us undergo a mechanization of our existence. This has resulted in the loss of communication between our body and mind. We use our body as a commodity and do not listen to its very deep and inner demands. The yogic practices presented in this book are designed for the present human need. Lest I be misunderstood, I would like to emphasize that I have changed nothing from the traditional concepts. I have presented the easier mental and physical exercises in slow progression. Taking the above example of language learning once again, I have split the words into letters and then put the letters back together again to make the words, in order to facilitate the learning of yogic practices. For example, if in a particular asana, neck and feet movements and breathing are involved, these three things are first taught separately. By this method, each of the body organs acquires flexibility independently before they get involved in a comprehensive effort. There are tremendous individual variations and each person discovers his or her weak points. My experience as a teacher has helped me to understand the

---

[2] *The word 'body' is used here in reference to the yogic tradition and it means our physical being, i.e., body, mind and intellect (*buddhi*).*

15

difficulties encountered by people during different practices. I have made it a point to note these so that the users of this book are not disheartened and will keep courage to proceed slowly towards success in various practices. Having overcome the weaknesses by repetition, the comprehensive movements and concentration become much easier for the learners. One acquires consciousness about the various parts of one's body and this disintegration is essential before beginning a search into the integration of the body as a whole and body and mind.

The yogic principles of Patanjali are widely spread and practiced by the Eastern gurus in the West. However, much to my distress, they are often mystified and superficially understood. Probably, the mystification and the over simplification are required to make them a saleable commodity in the West. One of the most famous schools of 'meditation' in the West has a tradition of doing its initiation ceremony for the newcomers with fruit, flower, cloth, etc., for the guru, like in the traditional Hindu initiation ceremony. When one goes for information to one of their centres, after explaining to you the details of the ceremony, they will tell you about the secret word you will be given after the ceremony and that by muttering the secret word you will attain salvation from all your troubles. "Why does this word have to be secret?" a friend of mine asked the initiator. "It has to be that way to attain meditation," he replied in a low voice and in a mysterious manner. Patanjali did not intend to make philosophy and practical training of yoga a mystery or a secret. In the second chapter of the Yoga Sutras, upon the practice of concentration, Patanjali states that svadhyana or muttering is one of the ways of achieving concentration. Answering the above question in its proper context, the word used to obtain a thought-free mind is kept secret because its repetitive pronouncement helps to push out all the other thoughts from the mind. Since the thought process works with associations, this particular word is kept to oneself, and thus remains free from association from other thoughts or thoughts about other people. For example, if one tells all one's friends about this particular word, then it is possible that at the time of muttering or japa, by the process of association, thoughts relating to these people will arise.

In this book, I take into consideration all aspects of daily living, body conditions and psychological states of our being. This book is not addressed to only a certain age group. It is never too early or too late to take the path which leads to self-realization. Some elderly persons might find it difficult to make some of the yogic postures described in this book, but they may benefit from other simple and fundamental yogic practices, pranayama and the practices for dissolution of thought. The sick and the bed-ridden can learn some simple yogic practices for fingers, hands, feet, etc. They can use concentration practices for self-healing and quick recovery. One should initiate children on the path of self-consciousness. At the end of the book, some special instructions are given for teaching yogic practices to children.

I request the users of this book not to treat it as an exercise manual and not to reduce yoga to only one of its multiple aspects. Please do read the first chapter carefully to understand the doctrine in its entirety before beginning to learn the fundamental practices presented in this book.

Vinod Verma
January, 1987

Acknowledgements

I wrote this book after I translated the *Yoga Sutra* of Patanjali to initiate people into adapting yoga as a way of life. I am grateful to my spiritual Guru, Patanjali who guided me to write this book.

I acknowledge my profound gratitude to my father from whom I learnt Yogasanas and the philosophy behind yogic practices. He took a great interest in my traditional education as well as providing me with an opportunity to study in some of the most renowned institutions of the world.

I am grateful to my two brothers for their enthusiastic participation for helping me with the illustrations and other related works for the book. My nephew and niece, Abhinav (6 years) and Gayatri (3 years) were absolutely adorable during the photographic sessions. Their devotion to learn Yogasanas and their enthusiasm for this book made it possible to include so many of their photographs.

Last, but not the least, I am grateful to my students from whom I learnt to see the problems in the path of yogic learning.

Health is the basis to attain virtue, wealth, sensuous pleasures and liberation whereas an unhealthy state destroys all this.

Charaka Samhita, Sutrasthana
Sixth century BC

Contents

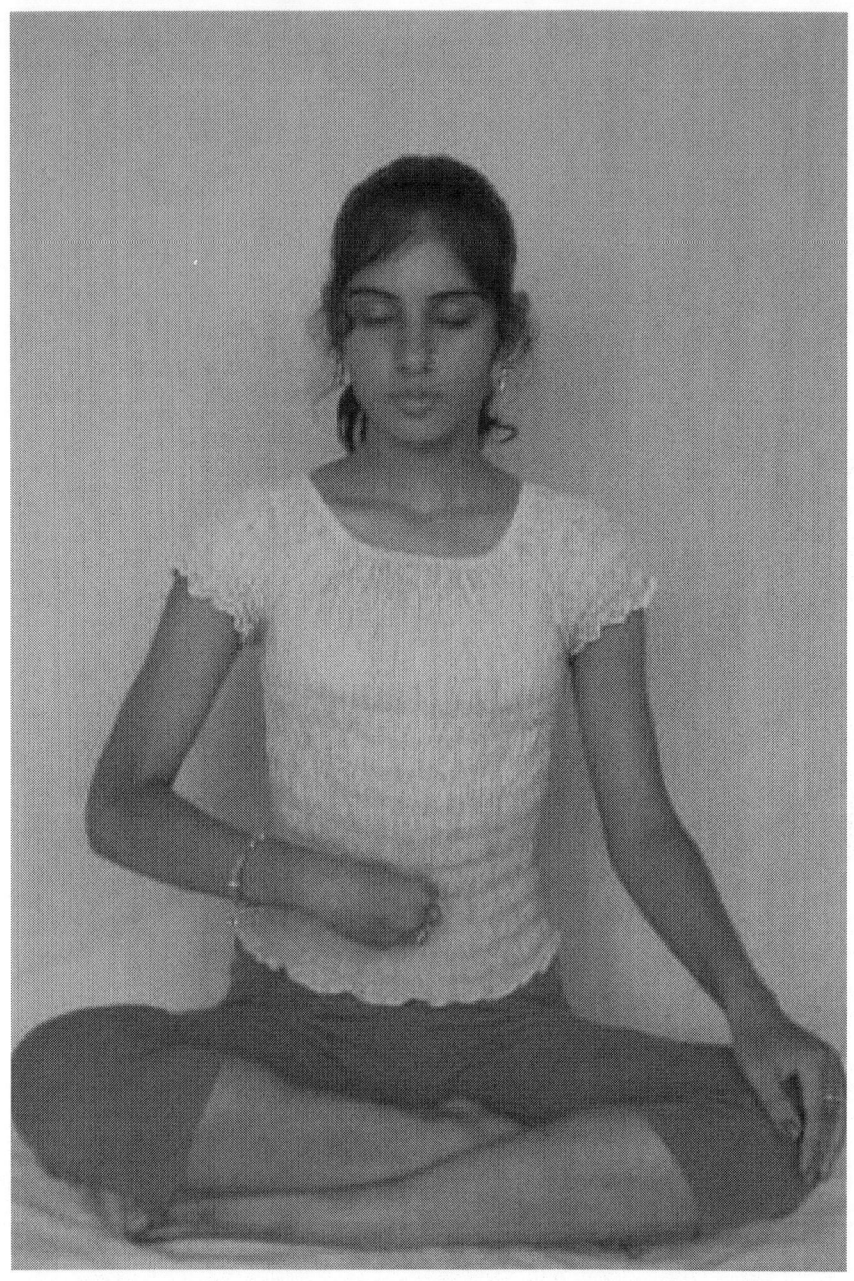

Chapter 1
Yoga and the Indian Tradition:
A Brief History

To know the history of yoga, we will have to go through 5000 years of Indian history. The first depictions of yogic practices were found on the seals and sculptures of the ancient civilization of the Indus valley which existed around 3000 B.C. In one of the seals, there is a prototype of the images of God Shiva, said to be the greatest yogi (*Mahayogi*). He is seated in a yogic posture surrounded by wild animals. God Shiva is also known as *Pashupatinath*, the protector of the animals and one of the very big temples of *Pashupatinath* is near Kathmandu in Nepal.

It is said that this civilization was subdued upon the arrival of Aryans from Europe and Central Asia around 2000 B.C. Aryans were mainly pastoral people who inhabited the regions between Eastern Europe and Central Asia. Indian scholars and some other well-known indologists do not agree to this theory of India's past. Somehow, it does not seem very rational to think that a great civilisation like that of the Indus, where extremely well planned cities were built and there was a very well organised society, was so easily plundered and destroyed by the, so called Aryans who were pastoral and without any known civilisation. Indus civilisation was at its peak, as there were established trade links with other major civilisations like Mesopotamia and Babylon. It does not seem rational to think that the nomadic Āryans became so brilliant in a short span of time to give to the world the great languages, timeless wisdom of the Vedas and other bodies of ancient Indian literature. (See more supporting documentation on this theme at Google Library: *The Scientific valediction of the Vedic Knowledge).*

It is interesting to trace the aetiology of the word "Hindu". The Indus River was called "Sindhu" by its inhabitants and because of the pronunciation difficulty, the neighbouring Persians called it "Hindu". This name came from Persia to Greece and became a universal name for the people of ancient India.[3]

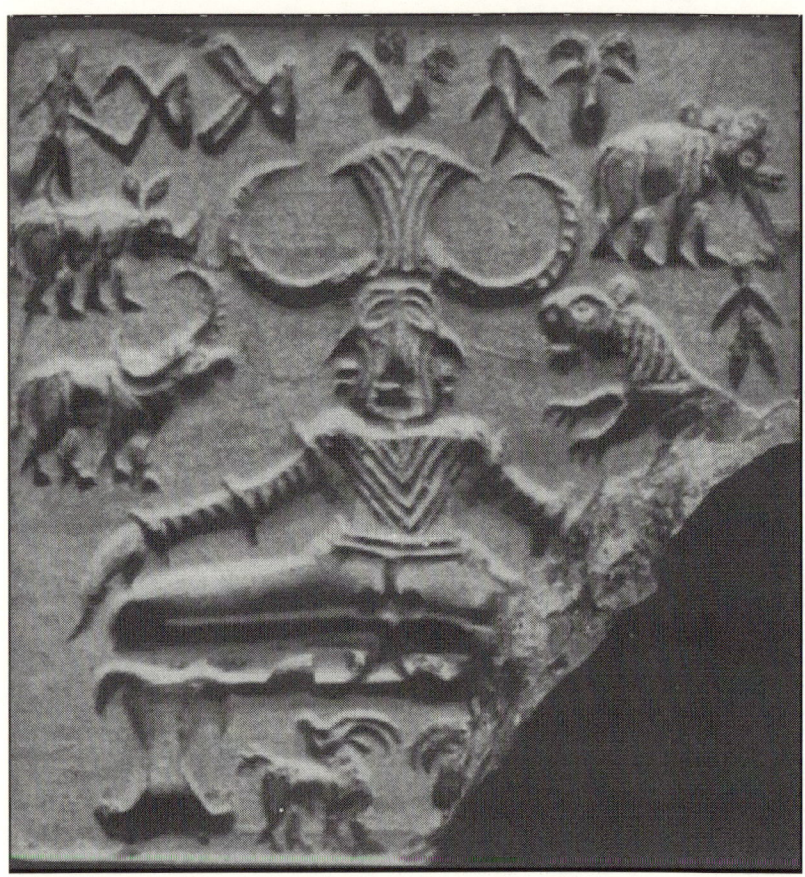

Figure 1: Prototype of Shiva sitting in a yogic posture, Mohenjodaro, 3000 BC

---

[3] *The words "Hindu Religion" or "Hinduism" are not used in this book because Hindu Dharma or Sanatana Dharma called so in Sanskrit, is not a religion but a Weltanschauung. It has no founder and it denotes the "eternal norm" or universal law. It has no beginning and no end. Dharma denotes the order governing the cosmos in all its manifestations: cosmic, religious, social, etc.*

24

Brahman—The Universal Soul or the Absolute

The western mind often becomes confused with numerous gods and multiple philosophies of the Hindu tradition. It is important to understand that all these gods were created to reach the ultimate reality— the Brahman or the Universal Soul or the Absolute. The different schools of thought originated to understand and realize the ways to reach the Absolute. The Brahman is un-embodied and it is difficult for the embodied to reach the un-manifested. The gods make this path easier. Secondly, the gods in their manifestations have philosophical symbolism. For example, God Shiva's trident is symbolic of three qualities of the *Prakriti* (these qualities are described on the following pages), his tiger skin represents desire, and his vehicle, the bull, is the four-footed Dharma. The goddess *Kali* represents power or *Shakti*. The garland of human heads around her neck symbolises wisdom and power and her red tongue signifies the power of *raja guna* - the quality which gives impetus to all activities. The sacrificial sword and the severed head held by her are the symbols of dissolution and annihilation. The girdle of severed hands around her waist signifies karma or action.

Vedas, Brahmanas & Upanishads are said to be written around 1500 B.C. However, their oral tradition existed much earlier than this period. These ancient texts prescribe methods of obtaining ultimate liberation from this world and to become one with the Absolute. Some centuries later, at the time of the great epic *Mahabharata*, this devotional and spiritual message was conveyed in the form of poems - the *Bhagavad Gita*.

Brahman is not God but the essence in all beings. In Bhagavad Gita it is described as:

The Supreme Eternal Brahman which can be called neither being nor non-being... , without any senses,

25

unattached, supporting everything, free from qualities and enjoying qualities,... within all beings, immovable and also movable, by reason of his subtlety imperceptible, at hand and far away is That[4]. Not divided amid beings; he devours and he generates. That, the Light of all lights, is said to be beyond darkness; wisdom, object of wisdom, by wisdom to be reached, seated in the hearts of all.[5]

A story in *Chandogya Upanishad* illustrates the incorporeal and immeasurable Brahman through the conversation between Sage Uddalaka and his son Svetaketu:

'Fetch me a fruit of the banyan tree.'
'Here is one, Sir.'
'Break it.'
'I have broken it, sir.'
'What do you see?'
'Very tiny seeds, sir.'
'Break one.'
'I have broken it, sir.'
 'Now what do you see?'
 'Nothing, sir.'

'My son, said the father, what you do not perceive is the essence, and in that essence the mighty banyan tree exists. Believe me, my son, in that essence is the Self of all that is. That is the Truth and that is the Self. And you are that Self Svetaketu!'[6]

The individual souls undergo a cycle of birth and death called *sansara*. From the deeds or karma of one life, the fruits in terms of pain and pleasure are decided for the next.

---

[4] *Often the pronoun "That" is used to describe Brahman and to emphasize its un-embodied nature.*
[5] Bhagavad Gita, *XIII, 12, 14-17.*
[6] Chandogya Upanishad, *VI, 12*

This cycle goes on and freedom from this pain of birth and death is sought. The freedom lies in following the path of immortality, that is, to become one with the Universal Soul or Brahman.

To grasp this idea of pain given by *sansara*, the cycle of life and death, we can illustrate it on a very brief time scale of one day. Imagine yourself being called into a room again and again and each time, after a very brief period (5-15 minutes) being told to leave. You leave just to be called back again. It is very boring, irritating and tiring. You will try your best to find means to stop it and will start inventing ways and means for that. On a larger time scale of several lives, each time we come to this world, we learn, build, get involved and attached to it as if we will be here forever. But one day, we have to leave and everything we built, loved and accumulated, remains as such. Our body, with which we identify ourselves, decays. The true self, according to the Vedic tradition is that essence of Brahman in us which goes away from the body at the time of death and is reborn. Ancient seers (*rishis*) sought ways to stop this "coming and going cycle" and to find eternal freedom and immortality.

This is an extremely brief background of the traditional Vedic concepts but nevertheless it gives a starting point for the comprehension of yoga as a path and as a philosophical discipline.

Yoga in the Context of the Hindu Tradition

The literal meaning of the Sanskrit word "yoga" is union, contact, connection or mental concentration. The word has its roots in the Sanskrit word "yuj" which means to yoke, fasten, join, unite, concentrate the mind or thoughts on, concentrate oneself or meditate deeply. The word "yuj" has common roots with the word "jungere" in Latin which means to join thus giving rise to the subsequent words as "yoke" in English, "joug" in French and "Joch" in German

27

(a frame by which two animals are joined for working together). The word 'yoga' denotes the path or the way which leads to the unification with the Absolute. It is also used to imply the exercises, bodily postures and other practices to obtain self-discipline.

Yoga is also one of the six great systems of thought or *darshana* of the Hindu tradition. These six great systems approach the aim of liberation from *sansara* in their own ways. Yoga is very closely related to another of these six systems- the *Sankhya*. *Sankhya* has provided a metaphysical basis to Yoga. Yoga in fact is a technical *darshana* which tells us the techniques to achieve the ultimate goal. Before we begin with the doctrine of Yoga, it is better to understand its metaphysical basis—the *Sankhya darshana*.

The *Sankhya* School of Thought

According to the *Sankhya* (the literal meaning of the word is 'number'), the process of cosmic evolution is divided into twenty-five components or *tattva*. *Purusha*, the Universal Soul and *Prakriti*, the Cosmic Substance are the two principal components. *Prakriti* has three constituent modes or *gunas: sattva* (modifications related to truth, virtue, beauty and equilibrium), *rajas* (modifications related to movement, force and impetus) and *tamas* (those modifications that restrain, obstruct and resist motion). *Prakriti* has no urge to action because it is inanimate. *Purusha* is the animating principle of *Prakriti* and it is without any qualities or *gunas*. It is that which breathes life into matter. It is only by the combination of *Purusha* and *Prakriti* that all existence manifests itself. By this combination, the next three components arise. They are: intellect, individuating principle and mind, thus, the individual identity. Through this latter arise five subtle elements (ether, air, fire, water and earth) and through these subtle elements arise five corresponding material elements (sound, touch, appearance, flavour and odour). Relating to these last five are the five senses (hearing, feeling, sight, taste and smell) and five organs of action (express, grasp, move, excrete and procreate).

Before the manifestation of the objective world, that is, before the association of *Purusha* with *Prakriti*, the three qualities of *Prakriti* are in a state of perfect balance. After the manifestation of existence, this balance is constantly changed by action (*karma*). *Karma* is the inherent nature of the combination of *Purusha and Prakriti.*

According to the *Sankhya* teachings, salvation lies in realizing the difference between the two ultimate realities of the cosmos through knowledge. The classical yoga of Patanjali is based upon *Sankhya* and we can say that yoga teaches us the practical aspects of the *Sankhya* wisdom.

The Yoga Sutras of Patanjali

Patanjali's Yoga Sutras or aphorisms, written around 500 BC are the first systematic treatise on yoga, which gave us not only the literary text, but also made yoga a doctrine or *darshana*.

The book consists of 195 sutras or aphorisms divided into four chapters. In this book, Patanjali brought together a series of ascetic and contemplative practices known in India from time immemorial and he has validated them from a theoretical point of view. Patanjali's greatness lies in his understanding of the working of the human mind and its analysis during various stages of concentration in the process of achieving meditation. Unlike the *Bhagavad Gita*, the central emphasis of the Yoga Sutras is not on devotion but on the individual himself along with his intellect, mind and body and their relationship to the cosmos.

In the first part of the Yoga Sutras, Patanjali defines yoga as "*Yogashchitta-vritti-nirodhah*", that is, "yoga is the hindering of the modifications of the thinking principle". The thinking principle of the mind is the constant flow of thoughts the mind undergoes. To stop this chain of thoughts by a conscious effort is yoga. Then he details the different types of modifications the mind undergoes and various means of hindering these modifications to attain steadiness of the mind. The soul, a part of the *Purusha* within us, is a passive observer of the modifications of the mind. When the modifications are stopped by meditation, the mind becomes identical with the soul.

Patanjali further illustrates different obstacles in the way of yoga and means to combat them. Then he outlines different stages of meditation. The highest stage of meditation leads to wisdom (*pragya*). Wisdom is to recognize the real self, the soul, as distinct from the Cosmic Substance.

The second part of the Yoga Sutras is about the practical aspects of yoga. Different means of attenuating afflictions are told. Afflictions are caused by ignorance or avidya. Ignorance lies in harbouring the belief that the material world and one's physical being are permanent. It is the inability to differentiate the soul from the Cosmic Substance. Further, Patanjali describes the eightfold yogic practices—the *Ashthanga Yoga* as a means of getting rid of afflictions. They are:

1. Forbearance.
2. Self-discipline
3. Yogic postures or asanas.
4. Pranayama or the controlled breathing practices
5. Restraint
6. Attention
7. Contemplation
8. Meditation

The third part deals with the last three yogic practices mentioned above: attention, contemplation and meditation and the accomplishments of these practices. When these three operate on one object, it is called *sanyama*. Through the practice of *sanyama* one develops a discerning ability and by performing *sanyama* on diverse factors, various *siddhis* are attained. A *siddhi* is a special psychic power like clairvoyance, ability to heal, etc. The *sanyama* is used for conquering the senses. A yogi has to be indifferent to his powers and ought not to exhibit wonders of his *siddhis* as this will ensue evil by his involvement in the worldly objects again.

In the fourth part, Patanjali describes that the *siddhis* are attained by birth, drugs, incantations of mantra, self-mortification or meditation. He clarifies that unlike the other *siddhis*, those obtained by meditation are not for the purpose of displaying. Instead, they are to be used for conquering the senses. Modifications of the mind are always known by the presiding soul which does not modify. The thinking principle, tinged by the soul and the object in question forms the totality of that object. The mind operates in association with the soul and exists for it in spite of being variegated by innumerable impressions. When the adept has got rid of impurities of the mind (afflictions) and has obtained discriminative knowledge, *viveka* i.e., the ability to distinguish soul from the Cosmic Substance, he/she is able to destroy previous impressions of the mind (*sanskara*) and results of the previous deeds (*karma*).

After having done this, the adept achieves *kaivalya* or the isolation of the soul from the Cosmic Substance. *Purusha* is bound to action because of its union with *Prakriti* and once they are isolated by the individual through yogic ways, the part of *Purusha* in the individual comes in union with the eternal *Purusha*. In fact, the individual soul is only separated from the Universal Soul as long as it is involved with *Prakriti*.

This is a brief description of classical yoga. I will refer to it as "the Yoga." It is also known as *Raja* Yoga (royal yoga) or *Rajadhiraja Yoga* (yoga of the king of kings). It is so called because through self-discipline, the mind becomes capable of ruling the senses. It does not mean that this form of yoga was used by the maharajas or kings as sometimes is explained in some modern books on yoga.

We will discuss several aspects of Patanjali's Yoga Sutras during the course of this book. But first it is important to know the other "yogas" one often hears about and their relationship to the classical yoga.

The Diverse Yogas

The three principle forms of yoga described in the *Bhagavad Gita* are: *Karma Yoga* (yoga of action), *Bhakti Yoga* (yoga of devotion) and *Gyana Yoga* (yoga of knowledge). *Karma Yoga* comprises of performing one's duty without attachment. The aim is to extinguish all desires for the fruits of one's actions. Action or *karma* is freed from the law of causality and does not constrain the individual to be reborn again. However, it is accepted that an absolute detachment from action is only possible through devotion. Lord Krishna says in the *Bhagavad Gita:*

He who performs his duties fully while taking refuge in Me, attains by the effect of My grace, the eternal indestructible abode.[7]

Gyana Yoga shows the path to liberation through knowledge. Knowledge here concerns recognizing one's

---

[7] Bhagavad Gita, *XVIII, 56*

true self (soul) and to see this 'self' as one with *Brahman*. But here also the aim is arrived at by the way of devotion.

He who sees a unity and worships Me abiding in all beings, that yogi lives in Me, whatever his mode of living.[8]

This devotion, however, is the devotion towards the Brahman or the Universal Soul as Krishna is a personification of Brahman.[9] The emphasis of the Yoga Sutras is more on personal effort than on devotion. The central subject is the individual himself along with his intellect, mind and body.

The fundamentals of the philosophy of the *Yoga Sutras* and that of the *Bhagavad Gita* are in *Sankhya* system of thought.

Children, not sages, speak of Sankhya & *Yoga* as different, he who is duly established in one, obtains the fruits of both.[10]

Patanjali's Yoga Sutras categorically describe the various stages of mental concentration and diverse ways to achieve the goal. The Yoga Sutras are religion-neutral and the word *Ishvara* (Part 1, Sutra 23) denotes no personified God but the *Purusha* or the Universal Soul of the *Sankhya*. It is said that:

A profound devotion towards *Ishvara* also (helps attain meditation). *Ishvara* is the Purusha, untouched by

---

[8] *Ibid., VI, 31*

[9] *The question arises why unembodied Brahman is personified. In this direction, it is said that the only way to convey the concept of Brahman to the masses is through personification. The pure philosophical conceptions are too 'dry' for a receptivity from the masses. Despite personification, the concept of Brahman is very clearly stated in* Bhagavad Gita *(see quotation 4). For a detailed evolution of this concept, readers are recommended J.Varenne's book* Yoga and the Hindu Tradition, *1976, The University of Chicago Press, Chicago.*

[10] Bhagavad Gita, *V, 4.*

afflictions, actions and their fruits and the consequent desires produced by these. In Him does the germ of omniscience become infinite. He is the Guru of (even) the earliest (created beings), as He is not bound by time. His appellation is *Pranava* (or the syllable 'OM').[11]

It is clear from all these sutras that the emphasis is on the *Purusha* which is symbolically expressed (Fig. 2) and not on a particular personified God.

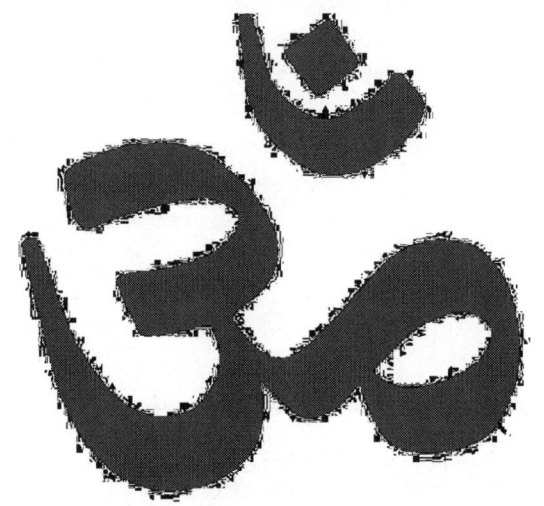

Figure 2: The syllable "Om", symbol of the Universal Soul

The purpose of the yogic practices is to destroy the impurities of the mind and to gain discriminative knowledge which leads to the recognition of the true self– the soul or a part of the *Purusha* within us. Table 1 summarizes the eightfold yogic practices described by Patanjali.[12]

---

[11] *Yoga Sutras of Patanjali, Part I, 23-27. This is author's own translation from her book on Patanjali's Yoga Sutras. The words in parentheses are added to make the comprehension easier.*

[12] *This table is also from my book on Patanjali. Space does not allow me to give greater details of Patanjali's eightfold yogic practices. Interested readers may refer to original literature like the* Yoga Sutra, Shiva Sanhita, Hatha Yoga Pradipika, Gheranda Sanhita, Yoga Darshana Upanishad

It is also worth mentioning here that the other doctrines and religions of India which did not accept the authority of the *Vedas* and were termed 'unorthodox' have also the same above-mentioned goal. Two such examples are Buddhism and Jainism.[13]

Concept of Body

Let us examine the concept of body in the Hindu tradition because in the present context, we are largely concerned with its well-being.

The body is like a chariot, the soul is its owner, the intelligence is its drive, the mind plays the part of reins, senses are its horses, and the world is its arena.[14]

The body, on the one hand, is the cause of involvement in this world and on the other hand, liberation is possible only through its efforts, thus designated as a chariot in *Katha Upanishad*. The body is pure because it houses the soul—a part of the *Purusha*. It can free the soul from the bondage of *Sansara by* doing a cooperative effort with the mind and the intellect. The body is the micro-cosmos of the macro-cosmos. We shall see in the following pages that in Tantric tradition, this idea is put very explicitly.

---

[13] *The founders of these two religions were two spiritual leaders of 6th century B.C.: Siddhartha, known as the Buddha and Vardhamana, known as the Mahavira. Jainism remained limited to India whereas the message of the Buddha was spread throughout Asia. Buddhism established itself as a religion 200 years after the* Nirvana *of the Buddha. It was spread in Asia through the efforts of a great Indian emperor Ashoka who reigned between 269 to 232 B.C.*
[14] Katha Upanishad, *III, 3*

Table 1. A summary of the Eightfold Yogic Practices or the *Ashthanga Yoga*.

1. Forbearance or *yama*	A. *Ahinsa:* or not killing or paining others B. *Satya:* veracity or truthfulness C. *Asteya:* not stealing D. *Brahmacharya:* continence, i.e., self restraint from yielding to impulse or desire E. *Aparigraha:* not coveting, i.e., not desiring for oneself the means of enjoyment.
2. Self discipline or *niyama*	A. *Shaucha:* purification • Phyical • Mental B. *Santosha:* contentment C. *Tapa:* austerity D. *Japa:* silent repetition of a mantra E. *Ishvarapranidhana:* a profound devotion to the *Ishvara*
3. Yogic postures or asana	The special postures devised for the purpose of yoga. They should become steady and pleasant with continuous practice.
4.*Pranayama*	*Pranayama* is the expansion of vital energy. Its practice involves a progressive deceleration of the respiratory rhythm and increasing the intervals between inhaling and exhaling and vice versa.
5.Restraint or *pratyahara*	*Pratyahara* is the indifference of the senses to their objects and their uniformity with the nature of the mind. Objects of senses are colour for sight and sound for hearing, etc.
6.*Dharana* (attention)	*Dharana* is fixing the thinking principle on internal space (*desha*).
7. *Dhyana* (contemplation)	*Dhyana* is a continuous state of *dharana*.
8. *Samadhi* (meditation)	*Samadhi* is when *dhyana* reaches a state where only the awareness of its meaning remains and even the personal identity is lost.

Note: *It is not possible to find the exact equivalent in English for the last three yogic practices. However, the tentative translation has been given in parenthesis. It is better to learn these words as such.*

Yoga and the Tantric Tradition

The word 'tantra' means to expand or to continue and in the applied sense it is that which extends knowledge. The word is also used as suffix to indicate any form of expanded literature which may or may not be a part of Tantric doctrine.

The Tantric principles and practices have had a tremendous influence on the philosophical and ritualistic traditions of India. They were also adopted by the Buddhists and the Jains. It is difficult to trace the origin of these practices but it is said that they go back to the Indus Valley civilization. The earliest codified Tantric texts date back from the beginning of the Christian era if not earlier.[15]

In Tantric tradition, *Purusha and Prakriti* are represented by the Lord and his creative power *Shakti.* They are considered as a God and a Goddess. In various schools the God is Vishnu or Shiva and the Goddess, his consort, Lakshmi or Parvati. Thus, the relationship between *Purusha and Prakriti* is in the form of male and female. The literal meaning of *Purusha is* male or man and the word *Prakriti* is of feminine gender. The human body is the micro-cosmos of the macro-cosmos and the existence is signified by the cohabitation of male and female principles. These are Atman and *Kundalini.* Atman (soul) is the part of the Lord (Brahman or *Purusha)* and *Kundalini* is the *Shakti* representing the Goddess or *Prakriti. Kundalini* literally means, "Coiled over itself". It is represented by symbols such as fire or serpent and it lies dormant in the human body. The aim of yoga is to awaken the *Kundalini.* The total isolation (*kaivalya*) of atman is achieved by the dissolution (*laya*) of the risen power of *Kundalini* into *Atman.*

---

[15] *A. Mookerjee and M. Khanna,* The Tantric Way, *page 10, 1977,New York Graphic Society. Boston.*

Within the human body lies a subtle body *(sukshma-sharira).* The subtle body is represented by a network of *nadis* or channels and it is compared to the universe itself. Various elements of the cosmos are represented in different parts of the body. *Prana* or vital air is guided into different parts of the subtle body through the network of *nadis.* The three principal *nadis* are *ida, pingala* and *sushumna.* Their intersections at six different places represent six of the seven major *chakras.* The literal meaning of the word 'chakra' is wheel but here it indicates the confluent points of vital energy for the rise of the *Kundalini.* The seventh chakra is on the top of the head and indicates the termination of the journey of *Kundalini* and its meeting with *atman.*

The tantric ways and symbolism form a part of the living tradition of India. The temples and the worship ceremonies have Tantric symbolism. Krishna with his consort Radha and the magic of his flute represent the *Purusha,* the *Prakriti* and the phenomenal world. *Shiva-lingam* in *yoni* pedestal symbolises the union of male and female organs in their cosmic totality. (Figure. 3).

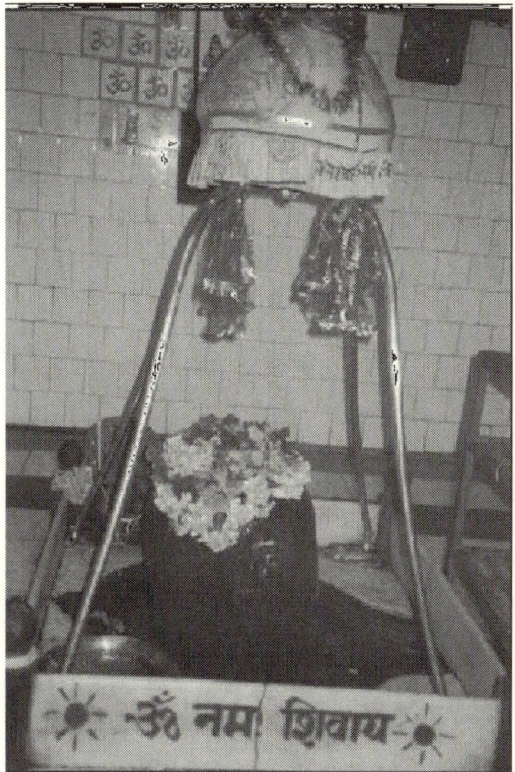

Figure 3: Shiva lingam and yoni

Influence of Yoga on Indian Life

It is worthwhile to examine the impact of yoga and the yogic practices on the day to day Indian life. Often Indians are faced with this question from foreigners, "Do you do yoga?" Most of the Indians would not know how to deal with this question and would say "no". From this, it is concluded by many that in modern day India, yoga is practiced by very few.

First of all, yoga is not something which one "does" in the sense of 'doing'—it is a way of life. Secondly, the Hindu mind is so deeply entrenched in tradition that yoga is an integral part of it. The names, definitions and intellectualisation of this philosophy are left to very few people as is always the case in any tradition. The impact of the Yoga philosophy is tremendous on the masses. *Karma, sansara, sanskara, klesha, atman, parmatman, maya* are words often heard in everyday life.

The Hindus are well aware of their final goal: the eternal liberation, and they are still more aware of the fact that this aim is very difficult to achieve.

As far as yogic practices are concerned, the most widely used is *japa*, that is, repetition of a word or a mantra given by a Guru or the name of a deity. This is a technique for the dissolution of thought. Some other yogic practices relating to the cleaning of the body are routinely done. Yogic practices are also used in combination with traditional medicine. When one visits a *Vaidya* or a traditional Ayurvedic doctor who has many generations behind him doing this profession (as is mostly the case), then one gets not only the medicines but also a long list of observances including some yogic and concentration practices for self-healing. Self-healing through concentration is also prescribed by the family Guru. It is a part of the oral tradition to prescribe and to know from each other asanas to cure various disorders and ailments. In the process of doing research on traditional medicine and travelling all over India, I discovered that an effort is being made to institutionalise the therapeutic applications of the yogic practices.

Finally, I would like to add that the yogic practices for health compiled in this book are not meant to be independent of the yogic philosophy. As is said earlier, 'health' in the present context is not meant for only physical fitness but for the harmony of 'our micro-cosmos' to the macro-cosmos. This is not done by doing yoga but by adopting the yogic ways. We have to learn to search and expand our inner resources by 'carrying out a churning operation within' ourselves using our own mind as the "churning agent" as said the *Upanishad:*

> **We know that milk is always the same colour,**
> **even though the cows that give it are of**
> **different colours; just so knowledge is one,**
> **even if the doctrines**
> **are diverse, just like**
> **the colour of the**
> **milk, even though the**
> **cows are different.**
> **And knowledge is hidden in the depth of**
> **each individual just as in milk the butter**
> **we cannot see is hidden;**
> **this is why the wise practitioner**
> **must carry out the churning operation**
> **within himself, employing his own mind**
> **without respite**
> **as the churning agent.**[16]

---

[16] Amritabindu Upanishad I, *18-20.*

Chapter 2
Yoga in the Context of Health: Mental and Physical Preparation

In the modern medical system, the body is treated like a machine which can be analysed in terms of its parts. This disintegration originates from a Cartesian dichotomy of the body and the mind. The modern mind is very much influenced by this dichotomy because the whole system of curing ailments, at least in the West, is based upon this ideology. However, in the present context, our starting point differs from this. The individual (body, mind, intellect and soul) is considered the micro-cosmos of the macro-cosmos. We, as beings, are an integral part of the whole and not we in parts make the whole. We are like glass balls in a jar with a narrow neck. One cannot move one ball without causing some sort of disturbance to the others. With this fundamental idea, the body is considered as an integral whole and the aim is to realize its unity with the mind through yogic practices. We have to search for this lost communication between the body and the mind. It is not something that has to be done by intellectualisation. It should come gradually through realization.

To appreciate a complete system, it is necessary to know the details of the individual aspects which make its entirety. It is essential to go through an experience of disintegration before beginning a search for integration. Let us discuss first various aspects of the vital factors sustaining the body.

The Body and its Sustaining Factors

The well-being of the body depends upon three principle

factors which sustain it. They are: breathing, eating and sleep. They are interrelated and interdependent.

Breathing: Technically, breathing is the alternate inspiration and expiration of air into and out of the lungs. It involves the exchange of oxygen and carbon dioxide between the atmosphere and the cells of the body.

In yoga, breathing is considered as the intake of vital energy and it establishes our connection to the universe. The vital energy pervades all organic and inorganic things. When breathing stops, our connection with vitality is broken and our body, with which we usually identify our 'self' ceases to be. Yet, how many of us consciously follow this vital process? A rhythmical deep breathing brings us in harmony with the universe. To bring our mind to this breathing process and to feel the air go in and out is very soothing. Breathing is quite rhythmical during sleep. By following one's breathing (or breathing consciously), both the body and the mind can relax. It is like partially imitating the state of sleep. One can also play different games with one's breathing by making it longer, shorter, giving short gaps between inhalation and exhalation, breathing fast as during running and very slowly as when one is completely relaxed and is just going to sleep. These are some preparatory exercises before beginning to learn yogic practices. You do not need special sessions for such exercises. They can be done at many different times such as before sleeping, while waiting, while taking a small pause from your deskwork and during so many other such situations. All you require for these exercises is your breathing mechanism and your mind. Do we not carry these two with us all the time?

Eating: We all know how vital food is for our existence. What we eat, how we eat and how much we eat play a very important role in our life. Long term wrong and excessive eating may cause dangerous and incurable illnesses. Fast eating and eating in stress gives rise to gastro-intestinal ailments. Such prolonged, minor ailments may one day translate into a disease in the organism.

We must learn to develop sensitivity to the effects of various foods we eat and to eliminate the foods that cause some sort of direct or indirect trouble to our system. The foods we eat should be varied and one should avoid eating the same things repeatedly. Too many fried and fatty foods should be avoided. Sweet foods like chocolates, cakes, etc., eaten in excess, are damaging to the teeth and to the digestive system.

Eating too much meat and lack of fruits and vegetables in the diet causes constipation and an imbalance of various elements in the body. Similarly, some meat-eaters resolve to eat vegetarian food and their lack of knowledge about a balanced diet without meat may lead to serious malnutrition. It is not recommended to change from being a meat-eater to a vegetarian drastically. One may begin the transition to vegetarian food from non-vegetarian very gradually and by carefully noticing the effects of this change on one's physical condition. If weakness or any other adverse effect is noticed, it should be discussed with a nutrition specialist or with your doctor.

Some people make it an obsession not to eat certain nutrients, because they have been told about their negative effects through mass media. They replace these nutrients with certain synthetic products. Sugar is a good example in this case. Two to three spoons of sugar per day in your warm drinks may do less harm than the synthetic products you use. It is better to avoid other products with sugar like biscuits, cakes, chocolates, highly sweetened cold drinks, etc., than to replace sugar with sweetening agents.

Overeating is dangerous in the same way as the lack of proper and sufficient food. Both extremes lead to malnutrition and disease. By excessive eating, the digestive system is activated and the body's eating capacity increases gradually. With time, this may cause the body to become overweight. Similarly, long intervals without food should be avoided. This inactivates the digestive system, decreases one's capacity to eat and thus, causes weakness. It is better to eat four times a day in smaller quantities than two big meals. A big meal after a long interval of not eating usually gives rise to a feeling of heaviness and laziness and a headache. Overeating, putting on weight followed by going on a diet is injurious for the internal organs. The digestive system is over activated first then it is suddenly deprived of its activity.

I will narrate an incident to illustrate how we can make ourselves ill by consuming excessive quantities of some foods or drinks. One of my neighbours always complained of pain in her stomach. She told me that her doctor did not understand the cause of her pain and the medicines prescribed gave her only a temporary relief. One day, this person invited me to have tea with her. She offered me a very strong black tea (big leaf Darjeeling tea). I asked her for some milk and sugar as this tea was too strong for me. She told me that she drank 1.5 to 2 litres of this tea every day. It was easy for me to understand the reason for her stomach troubles and it became possible to cure her.

Tea is astringent and acidic in nature. When taken in excess, it can cause stomach acidity and lack of appetite. To counteract this negative effect of tea, one should add spices like cardamom, cloves, cinnamon or ginger and the tea should be taken with milk and sugar. However, the high quality big leaf tea from Darjeeling has an exquisite flavour which is ruined by the addition of another flavour and taste. Tea should not be strong and not taken in large quantities.

46

Coffee, as a medicine is good to cure headaches, diarrhoea, mild fever and to cure the effect of alcohol and opium poisoning. However, taken in excess, over a long period of time, it may cause anaemia, weakness, insomnia, restlessness, breathing difficulties and chest pain. Some commercial cola drinks may have the same effect if they contain caffeine.

The process of eating should be slow and conscious. The food should be thoroughly chewed and while eating, one's attention should be on the process of eating. Food that has been quickly gulped down is difficult to digest because it lacks proper digestive juices which are secreted during the process of chewing. Avoid emotional outbursts of any sort during eating. Do not start eating when you are in an angry mood. Allow yourself five minutes and take some deep breaths to calm down before starting to eat your meal. In conclusion, get rid of anything which makes you tense before you begin to eat and bring your attention wholly to the process of eating. Meals taken in stress may do more harm than good to us by causing digestive disorders.

Sleep: Patanjali has defined sleep as "…that modification of the mind, which is maintained by the absence of new knowledge" (Part 1, sutra 10). It means that during sleep, the sense organs are inert and they are shut to any new external knowledge. Nevertheless, sleep is one of the modifications of the mind as it is a state of consciousness because firstly dreams are recalled, and secondly, even if one does not recollect events in dreams, one is aware of the state of sleep being good, bad or troubled. Sleep is a natural phenomenon like breathing, hunger, etc., and is temporally connected to nightfall. It is important for a good physical and mental state to have an appropriate quantity and quality of sleep. Excessive sleep makes one lazy and listless. It disturbs the equilibrium of the three basic qualities of nature in our body. Sleep is a state of stillness and is associated

47

with *tamas guna*—the quality that restrains, obstructs and resists motion. Excessive sleep causes an increase of *tamas* in the body and gives rise to various disorders. Similarly, lack of sleep makes one hyper excited and over active. It causes an increase of *rajas* in the body. *Rajas* is a quality which gives impetus and imparts motion. Thus, an appropriate quantity of sleep is very essential in producing an equilibrium or *sattva* state by balancing *tamas* and *rajas* in the body.

The normal sleep requirement for an adult is between 7 to 8 hours a day. Children and sick people need more sleep. During convalescence, more sleep is required.

We are all aware that sleeplessness and other sleep disorders trouble many people in our modern times and that the use of pharmaceutical products to cause sleep is very frequent in the western world. Lack of sleep or disturbed sleep gives rise to mental weakness, headaches, heaviness in the eyes, digestive disorders and pain and fatigue in the whole body. Sleep is a natural demand of our body and one often sees people sleeping at airports and railway stations in the most awkward sitting postures. Then why are some people not able to sleep even after a day's work and in their comfortable beds? The answer is very simple. It is due to unnatural ways of living that the natural phenomena of the body does not work the way it should. Consumption of drinks containing caffeine, a polluted noisy atmosphere, irregular meals, excessive worries are factors which may cause sleeplessness or some sleep disorders. One has to develop sensitivity to one's problems to find out what causes them. Taking a sleeping pill before going to bed is not a solution to the problem of sleeplessness or insomnia.

Sometimes the cause of this illness is very minor and one can help oneself with some changes in diet and lifestyle. Regular and balanced meals, regular evacuation, not talking too much at least one hour before going to bed, a calm sufficiently ventilated place of sleep and some yogic practices are recommended for people suffering from insomnia or breaks in a night's sleep. It is also recommended to have an early dinner and to do some yogasanas before going to bed. The topic of sleep will be discussed again with some individual yogic practices.

Some Observances for Yogic Practices

We have discussed the three major factors which sustain us. Now we will talk about some necessary observances which should accompany yogic practices.

1. *Yogabhyasa* (yogic practices) and *yogasanas* should not be done with a full stomach, full intestines or full bladder. The best time for most of the yogic practices is in the morning after evacuation. But if you cannot take time in the morning, then it is recommended either before dinner or 3 hours after any meal.

2. *Yogabhyasa* and *yogasanas* should be done in a quiet place, on a flat floor with a clean carpet or mat. Wall to wall floor carpet should be covered with a clean bed sheet or towel in order to avoid inhaling dust. One should wear loose or stretchable cotton clothes for yoga practice.

3. You should choose a large free space so as not to encounter hindrances during various movements.

4. It is best to do asanas in the open air if the climate permits.

5. Certain movements and postures tend to activate the salivary glands. The excess of saliva in the mouth should not be swallowed. It should be spat out. I have had difficulties with this, as students did not want to spit in the receptacles I had provided them. In yoga classes, spitting was somehow made a taboo whereas in a dentist's chair nobody paid any heed to

it. Why? Probably in people's minds yogic practices are associated more with a social activity than medical.

6. **Never** force yourself to do a movement or to make a certain posture. This way, you will do more harm to yourself than good. The body should be slowly made more flexible. The moment you feel uncomfortable with a particular stretch or posture, stop there. You will see that by repeated practice, you will attain success in making your postures more flexible and more comfortable.

7. **Stop** immediately a movement or stretching if you feel pain. Many of us discover some secrets of our body during yogic practices. For example, one person in a yoga class discovered that one of his legs gave him pain while he practiced leg postures. These weak parts of the body need special attention and their movements should be slowly increased by going slightly above the threshold each time.

8. Women should avoid doing *yogasanas* during menstruation. However, they can do *yogabhyasa* and concentration practices.

Minor Ailments and their Remedies

Let us see, first of all, what an ailment is and why such a malfunction occurs. We are constantly challenged by viruses, bacteria and poisons of various sorts and our body has a capacity to meet with these challenges. Different classes of blood cells build up the body's defence or immune system. They specifically destroy external attacks of infections or poisons. The immune system is capable of distinguishing external threats from normal tissue by recognising foreign molecules (antigens) and mounting a response that varies with the nature of the antigen.

Stress, fatigue, imbalanced diet, lack of sleep, lack of

physical exercise, dwelling in a polluted environment and lack of fresh air are generally the factors which make a normally healthy person vulnerable to external attacks by lowering the body's capacity to defend itself. The fight against a disease or an ailment consists principally of building up a strong defence system against attacking agents. It is a question of winning or losing against the external attacks. If we prepare ourselves with a strong sense of determination to win, we surely can! Consciousness of the self as a whole is a way to win. Each of us is different; we look different, we react differently and we behave differently. This variety is the beauty of nature. Through consciousness, we can know ourselves and protect ourselves better. No medical system that treats all human beings alike is ideal. It is up to us to know ourselves and to understand our problems before we subject ourselves to the caretakers of medicine.

The effects of various yogic practices and their therapeutic value will be discussed with the individual yogic practices. But before that, it is important to cure a few of the most common ailments.

Constipation by itself is a minor ailment, but if left unattended over a long period of time, may result in chronic headaches, haemorrhoids (piles), colitis, and various skin problems. Constipation is not only the infrequency of passing stool; it is also any kind of difficulty in passing stool. The stool should be neither too hard nor too fluid. Constipation is mostly caused by a sedentary lifestyle and lack of grains, vegetables and fruits in the diet. It may also result from a lack of fluid in the body. Some women have constipation a few days before menstruation and it may be accompanied by an attack of haemorrhoids for those suffering from them.

The simplest cure for constipation is to drink about half a

litre of hot water on getting up in the morning. Do not lie down again after drinking water; it is better to move around a little bit. The water should be either plain mineral water or clean drinking water which has been kept from the night before. Drinking water in the morning is a healthy practice for a general cleansing of the intestines as well as of the urinary system. One may make it a habit even without the problem of constipation.

A sore throat, the **common cold** and other minor virus infections in this direction are a few of the other common health complaints. Before any infection expresses itself fully, there is an incubation period. During this period our body is fighting against this infection and we feel tired. If we are sensitive and listen to the needs of our body, we can become aware of this process and can help ourselves to fight such minor infections. During and before the onset of such infections, one should get more sleep and take plenty of citrus fruits and herbal teas. Gargling, drinking Ayurvedic tea and taking 4–5 freshly crushed black peppercorns with honey are helpful in curing a sore throat and cough. *Pranayama* practices and cleaning of the buccal cavity and throat are of vital importance for curing a chronic bad throat and will be discussed later. Inhaling vapours from a mixture of citronella, eucalyptus, menthol and camphor or from commercially available balms containing such products helps fight larynx infections and opens blocked noses.

Minor pains: Pain in a particular organ or part of the body is a protest against the neglect or misuse of that specific part. The body has a perfected system and it has a way of warning us. When we treat it like a commodity, it protests. Taking pain killers in order to remove the pain is not a cure for pain. The most important thing is to find the cause of pain. One learns this by establishing a communication between the mind and the body. One must be indulgent with the areas affected by pain. The slightest pain should be attended to and taken care of. Headaches may be due to some digestive disorders, particularly constipation or stomach acidity. They may be also due to lack of fresh air, smoking tobacco and drinking beverages containing alcohol. Alcohol is known to cause stomach ulcers.

For immediate relief from pain, the external use of balms or pain relieving oils is suggested. Clove oil is very useful for relieving toothaches. Gargling with salt water is an additional help in this case. Wet heat, like a hot bath, is useful in muscular pains. Use of a hot water bottle in addition to pain relieving oils is recommended. Warm drinks like herbal teas, normal black tea with cinnamon, ginger and cardamom gives relief to minor pains and discomfort. The spices should be crushed in water first and then tea and milk (optional) may be added. One may sweeten the drink with candy sugar. Coffee also cures minor pains but it should not be made too strong because of its side-effects. The cure for various pains is also discussed with individual yogic practices. For chronic pains of unknown origin, it is better to undergo sophisticated medical examinations.

Fatigue is another major complaint of people in our times. It is prevalent particularly in big cities. It is caused by hyperactivity and excitement and by ignoring the body's need for rest, sleep and tranquillity. The simplest cure for fatigue is to attend to it and rest. 'Rest' means a complete halt of all activities and to get rid of the idea of 'doing something'.

In modern life, there is no real leisure. In some societies, doing various activities during your free time is considered very important. A fatigued person needs to stop such activities and needs complete relaxation. Relaxation does not mean only bodily repose; it is also the stillness of the mind. Reading a certain book of one's liking or listening to the music one appreciates, concentrates the mind and brings relaxation. It is important to remember that accumulative fatigue increases one's vulnerability to various infections and to control fatigue is in our hands.

Yoga—A Way of Life

The practice of yoga is not only limited to a half an hour session every day. It begins early in the morning with our getting out of bed. Most of us get up in a hurry. Many of us jump out from our beds, rush to the bathroom in order to get ready and begin our daily routine. We brush our teeth and take a shower etc. We should ask ourselves this question. "Am I with myself during all this time?" What does one mean by "being with oneself?"

We are practically never alone. In spite of being physically alone, we fill our rooms, apartments and houses with crowds of people or we go out with other people in our thoughts. To illustrate this point, here is a little story from the Buddha's life. Once, two disciples of the Buddha (monks) were walking near a lake when they heard cries of a drowning woman. The monks were not supposed to touch a woman. The question came whether these two disciples should break this rule or be so cruel as to let the woman drown. One of the disciples decided to save the woman; he jumped into the water and brought her out. When the monks reached the ashram, the other disciple complained to the Buddha about his companion touching a woman and bringing her out of the water. The Buddha replied, "Well, my dear fellow, your companion brought the drowning woman out of the water and left her at the bank of the lake. You carried that woman with you all the way back and brought her to the ashram."

The mind is very fast moving. The thought process works in a chain and this chain continues throughout our life– just like the heartbeat and other vital functions of the body. It is only through the mind that we can control the mind. The first step consists of being aware of our thoughts and then next is controlling them. This exercise begins as soon as we get up. Instead of bringing crowds with us, we should try to be with ourselves.

When you wake up, try and begin to think about your whole body, its substance in material terms and the space it occupies on the bed. Your mind should follow the actions of your body. The next step is probably getting out of bed and going to relieve yourself. Think about this process and about the feeling of relief you get from it. Brushing of teeth should be followed equally with all your attention. Are you cleaning your teeth with care and from all sides? Both rows of teeth have six surfaces. Are your gums alright? Is your buccal cavity clean? Is your tongue clean?

Just think how many of us know in detail the shape of our body, the shape of our feet, toes, nails, etc. Begin to know these, while taking your shower or bath. Some of you might think by now that all this is too much as you are in a hurry every morning and you have no time to "be with yourself". It is a mistaken notion. You do not need extra time for the above-described exercises. It is only diverting your mind from other people from outside and bringing it home to yourself.

We have mirrors to look at our external appearance. Besides, the others around us mirror our outward being. If you have a spot on your face and are unaware of it as you go out, the looks of the passers-by will make you realize soon that there is something wrong. But most of us do not try to mirror our inner being. We are unaware of our inner wealth and power and do not explore it because, we have had no exposure or training to do so. Learning in this direction begins with these small exercises of following our thought process and making an effort to concentrate our thoughts on the activity we are involved with at that particular moment– it may be the most mundane activity of our daily routine. Thus the practice of yoga begins with our effort to be with ourselves.

Chapter 3
Yogic Practices (Yogabhyasa), Yogic Postures (Yogasanas) and Concentration Practices

I have divided various yogic exercises and asanas to cover a time period of 9 weeks. But you need not follow the prescribed time period and may take four weeks or more to accomplish one week's programme. You have to develop your own feeling for time, taking into consideration the demands of your body and mind. Every person is different; some are more stiff than others, some have already had experience and training in related fields, some regularly exercise and do sports whereas others lead a rather sedentary life.

As has already been mentioned, one should not force oneself while doing a yogic exercises or asanas. The way to learn a difficult posture is by little but regular practice. As is relevant for any kind of learning, it is more beneficial to make a daily routine of practicing. With lengthy time breaks, the body loses its acquired flexibility and one has to begin from the beginning again. In each week's programme, there are four to five different yogic practices, and learning them well opens a way for subsequent more difficult and complicated asanas and concentration practices. It is advisable not to proceed to the next week until you have mastered the previous week's programme and feel at ease with those yogic practices. The body gradually relaxes with repeated practice and the accompanying breathing rhythm. Yogic practices demand your total attention to harmonize the body movements with breathing. They form an integral system giving exercise not only to muscles and joints but also by revitalizing the internal organs. Thus, yogic practices deal with all the intricate details of human anatomy and provide equilibrium to the body and the mind.

FIRST WEEK

A. Warming Up the Body by Pressing and Rolling

The mind has very wide horizons and wanders very quickly to distant places, people and things. We start with the basics and try to reduce the horizon of the mind with the following exercise.

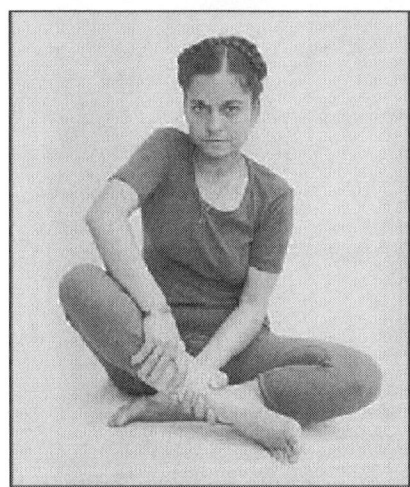

Figure 4 *Warming up*

Sit down in a comfortable and relaxed posture. Make sure that your neck and shoulders are not tense. Check that you are sitting straight and your vertebral column is not curved. Start pressing one of your feet with both your hands and move upwards slowly (Fig. 4). Go around all sides of your leg with your hands applying continuous pressure

Concentrate on the parts of your body you are pressing. Continue pressing your leg upwards till you come to the pelvic joint. Commence with the other leg in a similar

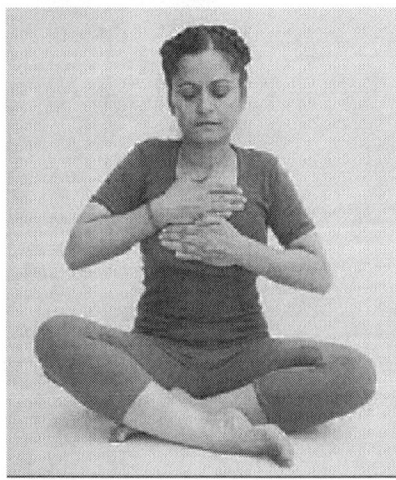

Figure 5 *Warming up*

58

way. The next step is to press your one hand with the other and to go upwards to your shoulder, to the side of your neck and to your head. Repeat this process with the other hand on the other side of your body. Now with both hands fully open, press your abdomen with a slight pressure, move upwards to your thorax (Fig. 5), and from there to your neck and your face to the top and back of your head and neck. By 'pressing', in this way, you will realize that you have touched, pressed and felt nearly all parts of your body except your back. The next practice deals with the back

Lie down on your back. Bend your legs and bring them to your chest Put both your arms around your bent legs and clasp your hands together. Now, lift your head up towards your

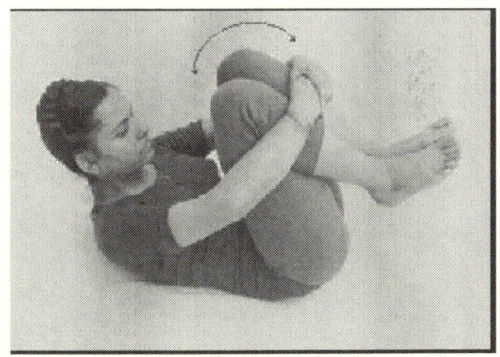

Figure 6 *Warming up*

knees and rock your body for-wards and back-wards (Fig. 6). This will give a soothing feeling to your back. Repeat 5 to 6 times. The next step is to make the same posture

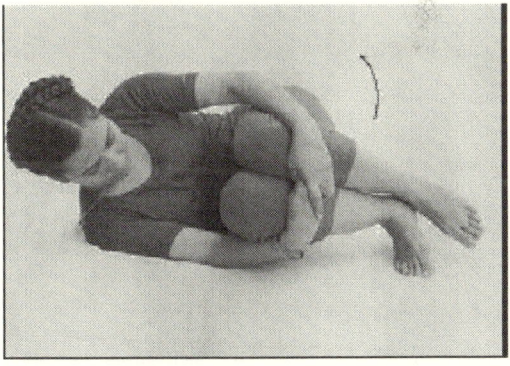

Figure 7 *Warming up*

but to roll the body sideways (Fig. 7). Repeat this also 5 to 6 times.

Benefits: Pressing and rolling tone up the body and enhance blood circulation. It helps to stop the mind from wandering and helps you to concentrate on your body.

B. *Shavasana* or the Dead Body Posture

Shava in Sanskrit means dead body. This asana consists of imitating a dead body, i.e., loosening your body organs to bring yourself to a complete state of relaxation. As easy as it may sound or appear in the picture (Fig. 8), 1 would like to warn you that it is quite difficult to achieve a state of complete relaxation. The process of inducing relaxation may generate tension. So please take it easy. Do not say to yourself again and again, "I must relax! I must relax!" There is a technique for relaxing which makes this process natural and spontaneous.

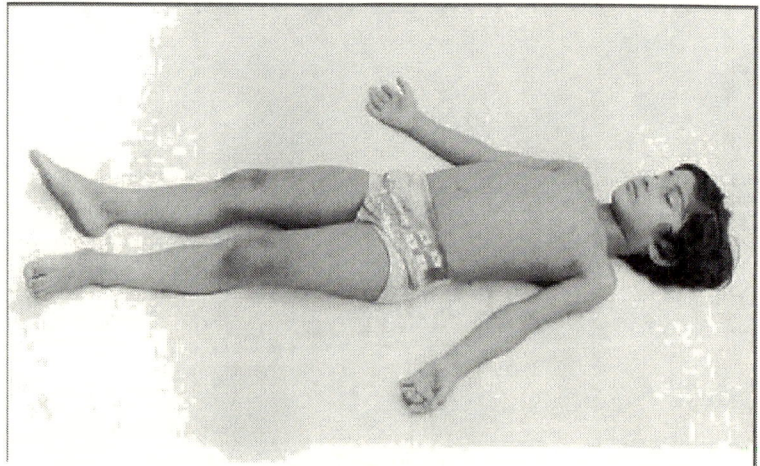

Figure 8 *Shavasana*

Lie on your back with your hands and feet apart and palm upwards (Fig. 8). Close your eyes. See to it that your shoulders and neck are relaxed and your forehead is smooth and free from a frown. Once you feel well adjusted with all parts of your body, start thinking about them in detail. Bring your thoughts to one particular part of your body, for example, the right foot. Start imagining how your foot looks and then bring your thoughts to your ankle. Proceed in a similar way as you have done for pressing but this time only with your thoughts. In this case, you are visualizing the form and appearance of your body rather than feeling it through the sense of touch. Imagine that all parts of your body are gradually getting heavier. Feel this heaviness in all parts of your body individually. Accompanied with this feeling of heaviness, your breathing will also get slower. Stay in this asana from 2 to 4 minutes or as long as it feels good. Get up slowly from it.

Benefits: This asana is particularly good in helping one to relax and in controlling tension and insomnia. It is recommended between long hours of work if one feels fatigued. It revitalizes the whole body.

Suggestions: This asana is very beneficial for old people who often have problems sleeping continuously throughout the night. It is also suggested for the sick and the bed-ridden to help promote mental relaxation. People, who are nervous by nature or those who lead rather hectic lives can benefit a great deal from this asana. It is particularly recommended for people in high positions such as managers and others who suffer from a similar amount of stress.

C. *Yogabhyasa* (Yogic Practices) for the Hands, Fingers and Feet

Hands

This practice consists of making circular movements with the hand from the wrist. The forearm provides an axis to the movements of the wrist and the hand while the elbow stays in one place.

Pre-exercise: Sit down in a comfortable posture. Rest your elbow and a part of your forearm on your knee. Bend your hand forward from the wrist as far as you can. Repeat this movement by bending your hand backward and sideways. The next step is to make circular movements with your hands from the wrists as if you are making circles in the air with your forehand. If your elbows stay in place and movements involve principally your wrists, then you have understood the basic aspect of this practice.

Yogabhyasa: Stay seated in the position described above. Relax and take a few deep breaths. Now start the above-described movement slowly (Figs. 9, 10). Do not tense up your hand and keep your fingers spread out. Now close your eyes, try to concentrate on the movements of your hand and feel how this movement involves several muscles of your fore- and hind-arm and how it makes the wrist and elbow joints work. You may do the movements with both

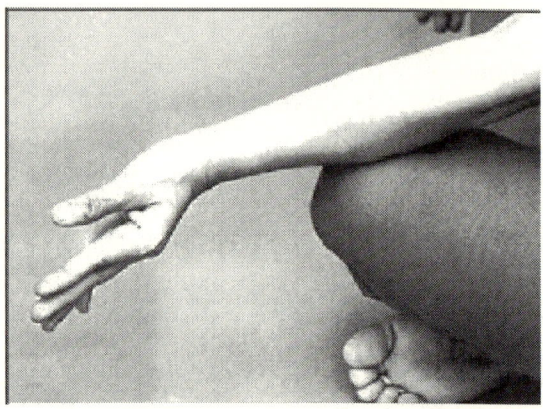

Figure 9 *Finger yoga*

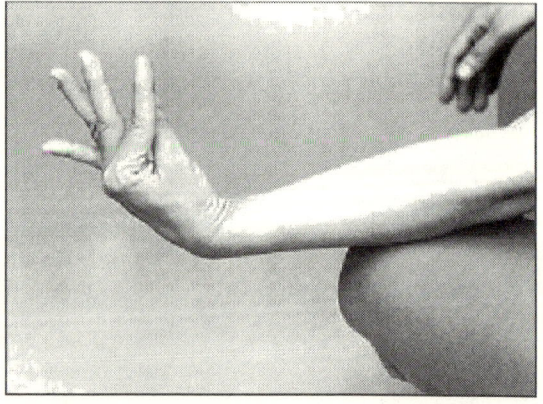

Figure 10 *Finger yoga*

hands simultaneously. The two important factors are: 1) to do the movements very slowly, and 2) not to stiffen up your hand and wrist. Repeat 8 to 10 times and then take a rest for a few breaths. Repeat the same movements by changing the direction (clockwise to anticlockwise or vice versa).

Benefits: This practice gives exercise to the wrist joint, elbow joint and hand muscles. It also energizes some muscles of the fore- and hind-arm.

Fingers

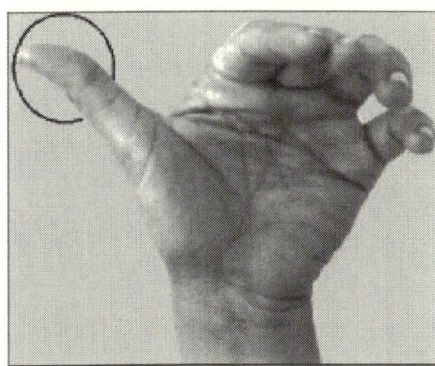

Figure 11 *Finger yoga*

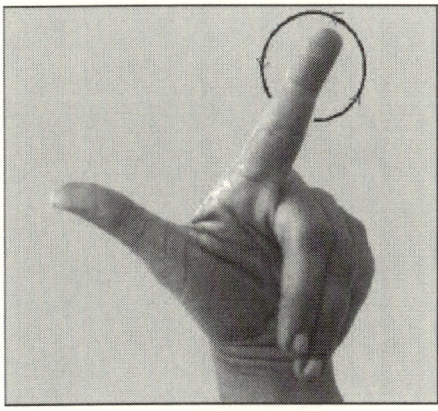

Figure 12 *Finger yoga*

Stay seated in the same position as for the previous practice. Do the same round movements with your thumb and then successively with each of your fingers (Figs. 11, 12). This movement is done from the base of the thumb or fingers. Keep the pace of the movement slow. You will notice that it is easier to do this practice with the thumb and the index finger than with the other three fingers. This is because the muscles and joints of these fingers are not often used for these special movements. Repeat this exercise only a few times the first day, as it is

63

tiring. Try to concentrate and realize that many muscles of the hind and forearms are involved in these movements.

Benefits: This practice strengthens the fingers and is good for the nerves. Probably some of you are aware of the Chinese therapy through hand massage. This practice is similar. It is also good for the heart muscles. It is particularly beneficial for people who work with computer keyboards. It is a precautionary practice against finger arthritis.

Suggestions: This is one of the yogic practices that you can do on a bus, tram or train, waiting for a doctor, a lawyer or a client, or during any other such situation. Use your time beneficially!

Feet

This practice is quite similar to the one described for the hands. Here, similar movements are made with the ankle, and circles in the air are made with the forefoot. The knees and legs stay still except for a small accompanied movement of the foreleg around its axis.

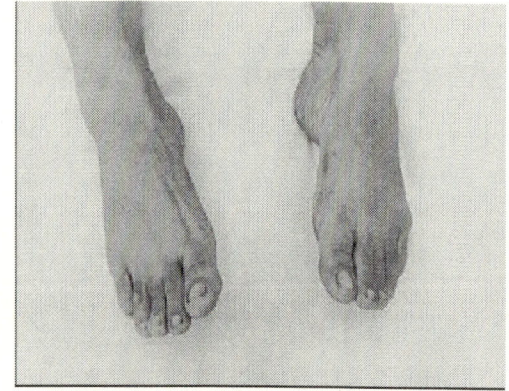

Figure 13 *Feet yoga*

Figure 14 *Feet yoga*

Pre-exercise: Lie down on your back. Keep a distance of about 30 centimetres between your feet. Stretch your feet outwards as far as you can. Repeat the same by

64

bringing them forwards and then towards right and left successively. Try to feel the effect of this stretching on your leg muscles and your ankle and knee joints. Now, make circular movements from your ankles so that your forefeet make circles in the air.

Yogabhyasa: Relax and loosen up your body. Concentrate on your feet. Stretch them outwards. Start making round movements as described above by first going towards the right and ending the circle coming back from left, i.e., moving in a clockwise direction (Figs. 13, 14). The movements should be slow and smooth. After finishing one circle, relax for two to three breaths and repeat the circle again. Take a longer pause (10 to 15 breaths) before repeating the same movement anti-clockwise.

When you feel confident enough with the feet movements, begin to synchronize each movement with one breath. Begin the movement and start inhaling slowly and smoothly. Half way around the circle, begin to exhale slowly. Exhaling and completion of the circular movement should terminate at the same time. Air should not be breathed in and out too quickly. Harmony between breathing and the movement comes with practice. Give yourself time and do not tense up if it does not work right away.

Benefits: A very healthy practice for people who wear closed shoes or high heels. It is very soothing for tired ankles. It also exercises the knee joints and leg muscles, particularly the dorsal muscles of the fore and hind leg.

Suggestions: Hands, fingers and feet movements are specially recommended for people who have restricted physical activity because of illness and some other reason. These three yogic exercises are beneficial for revitalizing stiffened wrist and ankle joints and muscles after an accident. However, they should be gradually adopted in

65

order not to cause an injury to the recovering parts.

D. *Uttanapadasanas* or the Raised Leg Postures

There are four different asanas in this series. The first consists of lying down on the back and raising one leg at a time and the second involves raising both legs together. The third and the fourth are like these two asanas respectively but are done while lying on the stomach.

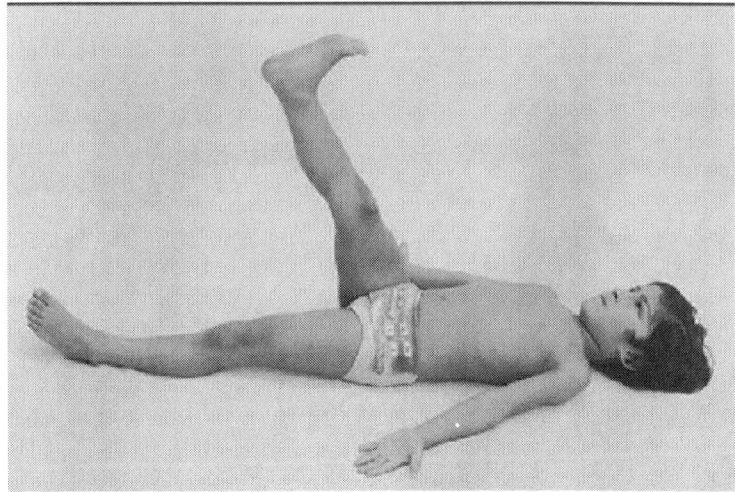

Figure 15 *Uttanpadasana*

a. Lie down on your back as you did for *shavasana*. Relax, take a couple of deep breaths and begin to concentrate on your right leg. Then slowly lift the entire leg up while inhaling. Take it as far as you can and stop at the point of your limit (Fig. 15). Hold your breath at this moment. Then, slowly bring your leg down while exhaling. Put the leg on the floor very gently. The knee should not be bent in this asana and the force should come from the thigh. The entire leg should be in a straight line. Your thoughts should follow the movement of your leg and the rhythm of your breathing. These two should be harmonized. After doing this movement once with the right leg, give an interval of a few breaths and repeat the same for the left leg.

b. The second asana of this series involves raising both legs. Bring your legs together so that your feet are touching each other. Raise both legs together (Fig. 16). Breathing and other instructions are the same as for the previous asana. Take care that in these asanas, your neck and arms do not move. Your shoulders and the upper part of your back should be relaxed. You should not bend your knees and that your movements are very slow. Your mind should concentrate on harmonizing the movements of your legs with your breathing. Inhaling and exhaling should be smooth and slow.

c and d. These two asanas are the same as the previous ones but these are done lying down on your stomach (Figs. 17, 18).

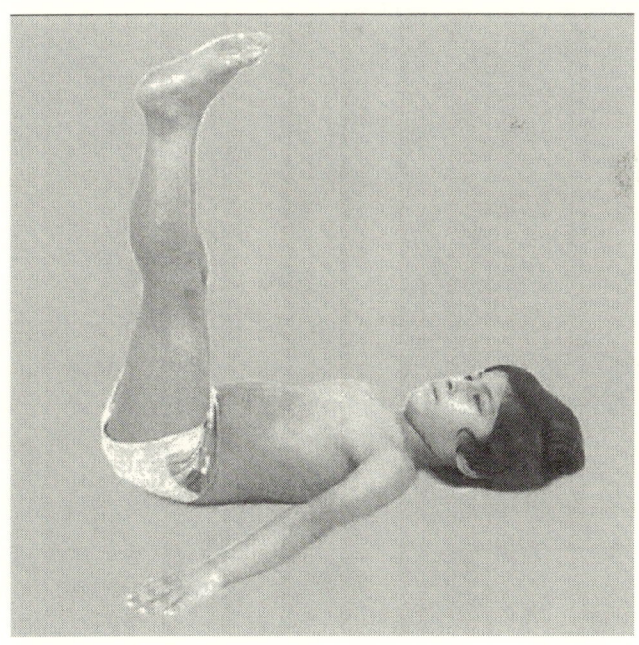

Figure 16 *Uttanpadasana*

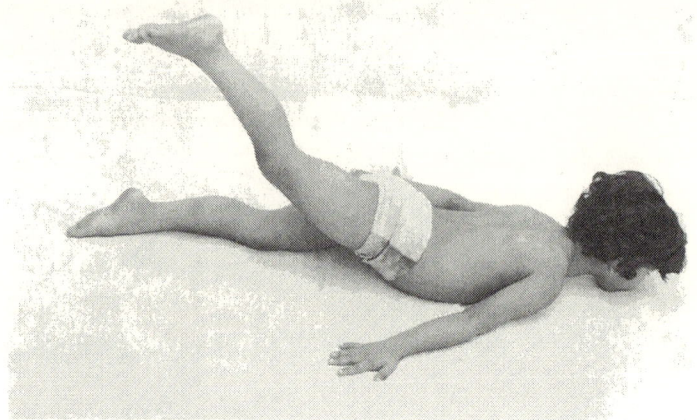

Figure 17 *Uttanpadasana*

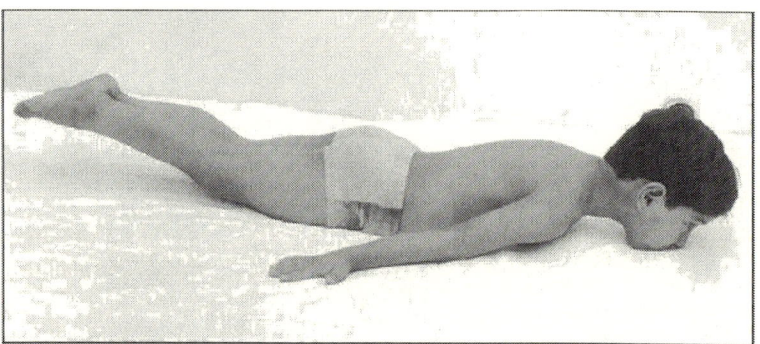

Figure 18 *Uttanpadasana*

Possible difficulties: Some people might discover that one of their legs is weaker than the other. They may experience some pain while raising their leg. There could be various reasons for this. The pain or discomfort in the leg may be due to muscular weakness; a defect in the pelvic joint or it could be of some nervous origin (neuralgia). It could also be due to the difference in the length of the two legs. These asanas can help to make the weaker leg stronger. But they should be performed with great care and indulgence for the weaker limb.

Benefits: Asanas 'a' and 'b' give exercise to the pelvic joint, to the abdominal muscles and are especially good for the intestines and the stomach. They are helpful against constipation and help to increase appetite. They are useful in reducing paunch and strengthening the abdominal muscles. The asanas c and d energize the muscles of the hip and the lumbar region and also give exercise to the lumbar vertebrae. They are also good for the superficial abdominal muscles.

The most important therapeutic value of these four asanas is for curing sciatic pains. However, for the treatment, these asanas should be done regularly over a long period of time. Two factors that trigger sciatic pains are fatigue and an exposure to cold. Proper rest should be taken and the body should be kept warm. The therapy should be aided by the application of balms or pain relieving oils on the sensitive area.

Caution: These asanas require a tremendous effort of nearly the whole body up to the neck and the head. It is easier to make the upward movements with the legs at a faster speed but raising the leg/legs slowly and then staying in the posture and coming down slowly involves not only the muscles and joints but also the abdominal internal organs. Do these asanas only a few times in the beginning and gradually increase the number of times. Do not do these if you feel tired or unwell.

SECOND WEEK

A. Reflections on the Previous Learning

The next step of learning yogic practices begins by self-examination of the previous learning. Are you at ease with the practices learnt until now? Does your breathing harmonize with your movements? You should not be inhaling and exhaling in jerks. Breathing should be slow and regular. Beginners encounter two major problems. The first is that most people have difficulty in loosening up. They remain stiff and their muscles and vertebral column remain tense as if they were "on the alert". This probably is a phenomenon of our modern civilization and this state is due to a hectic lifestyle, having constantly the idea of doing something and seeking for more and more material goods and luxuries. Everybody must do everything very fast and nobody has time. Sitting, thinking, relaxing and being conscious of ourselves and the universe we live in are somehow down-rated thoughts. "How to gain consciousness?" is also sought in organized institutions and falls in the category of "doing something". We have forgotten probably the most simple thing of life –just to be, to be ourselves.

The second difficulty which people often face in the beginning of the yogic practices is with the pace of the movements. One tends to move individual parts of the body faster because it is easier. While doing yogic practices, one has to remind oneself again and again to go very slowly. We are not used to such slow movements during the normal course of life.

B. Cleaning of the Mouth, Buccal Cavity and Throat

Those of you who have been to India may have heard an orchestra of many sounds Indians make while cleaning their mouth, throat, etc; during the early hours of the morning. After reading this page, you will probably join this orchestra. This cleaning should be done in the morning before having eaten anything and about 10 minutes or more after having drunk your hot water.

First of all, brush your teeth properly taking your brush in all the three directions of the upper and lower rows of your teeth and reaching all the far away corners. Then rinse your mouth properly several times. It is important, specially these days, when we know that many of the toothpastes contain toxic substances like sodium dodecylsulphate which dissolves the cell membranes and ultimately causes decay in the teeth rather than protecting them. Then, after having rinsed your mouth well, stick your tongue out and clean it softly with your toothbrush. Rinse your mouth and repeat this process of cleaning the tongue 2 to 3 times. Now stick your tongue as far out as you comfortably can and tickle it with your brush or fingers. There will be a noise from the deeper part of your throat, you will cough a little and some saliva will come out from the mouth. Simultaneously, the stomach is temporarily retracted. Spit out the extra fluid from your mouth and rinse again. Those of you, who have drunk water before, may vomit some water. If your stomach is healthy, this vomited out water will have no smell or taste. But if this water is bitter, sour or smelly, it is indicative of an unhealthy stomach. In classical yogic language, this practice is called *Jala Dhauti*, which literally means "purification by water" and comprises of drinking salted hot water and then vomiting it out. For doing this practice, drink about ¾ litre (3 cups) of hot and salted water and vomit it out after a few minutes by tickling the deeper part of your throat with your fingers. For vomiting, bend not more than 90° in order not to put any pressure on the abdominal part. The maximum number of the vomiting impulse should be eight.

Benefits: These cleaning practices are healthy for the care of the teeth, gums and stomach. They remove bad smells from the mouth. They activate the salivary glands and ensure their proper functioning, and remove minor infections from the throat. *Jala Dhauti* provides exercise to the stomach, ensures good digestion and removes acidity.

71

Suggestions: These practices are particularly recommended to those who have a frequent sore throat. However, they should also take the precautions and treatments prescribed in the previous chapter for the same. Jala Dhauti is also recommended to people who have a sensitive stomach.

C. Asanas for the Jaw Bones and Jaw Muscles

In Figs. 19 and 20, three-year-old Gayatri might seem to be teasing another child by sticking her tongue out in two different fashions. But these two postures perform quite a complicated task. Musculature around the mouth, jaw and chin is quite complicated. For example, the muscles of the upper and lower lip are horizontal to the lips and from the side of the mouth where they join; three different muscles originate in different directions. I do not want to go into anatomical details; my idea is to make you feel the muscles rather than to learn about them. Such a simple posture, like sticking your tongue out, gives exercise to and energizes not only the musculature around the mouth but also the jaw bone and joint.

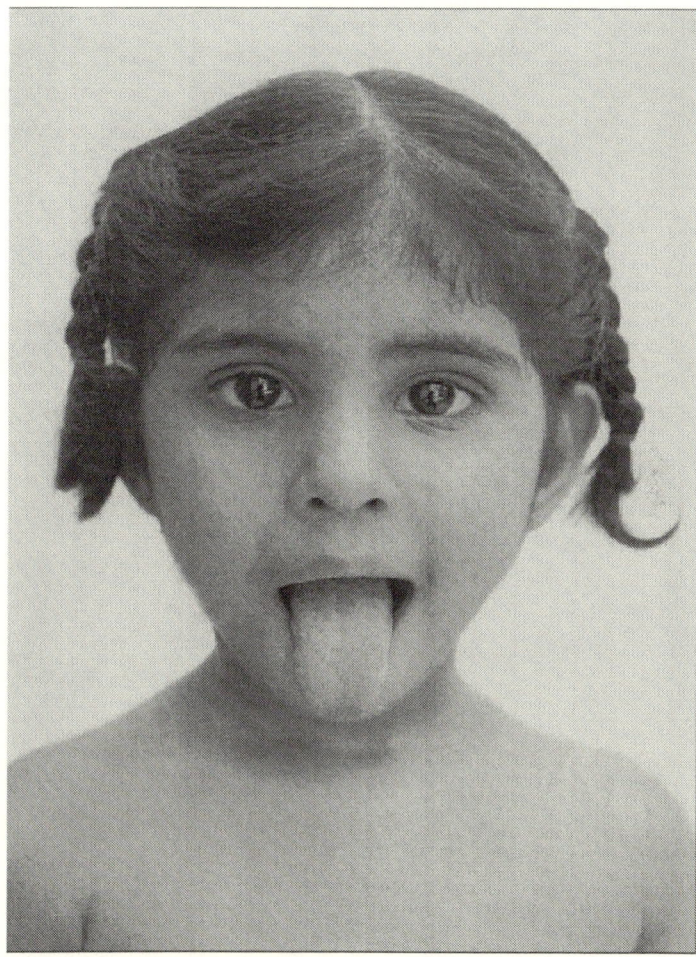

Figure 19 *Jaw and Tongue Yoga*

These asanas are very simple. For the first one, stick out your tongue downward to your chin as far as you can (Fig. 19). Do not force yourself to go very far out with your tongue as you might hurt your jaw muscles and get a cramp. Gradually your capacity to stick out the tongue farther will enhance. Stay in this asana only 15 to 20 seconds and repeat it 4 to 5 times.

In yogasanas, various movements are balanced by counter movements. Here is the first example of this. The next asana consists of sticking the tongue upwards to the nose (Fig. 20). Do this in a similar way as you did for the previous one.

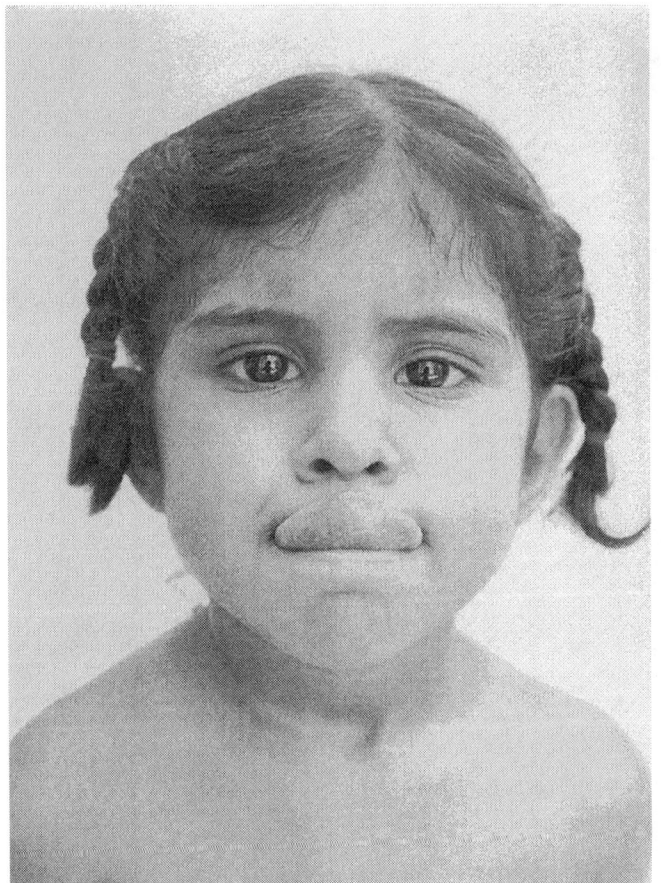

Figure 20 *Jaw and Tongue Yoga*

Benefits: These two asanas energize the tongue and a part of the face muscles and give strength to the jawbone joints.

Suggestions: Children love to learn these asanas and one can initiate them into yogabhyasa by teaching them such practices which they find amusing at the same time.

D. Asanas for the Neck

I have chosen two asanas in this series which provide movements in two different directions for the cervical vertebrae.

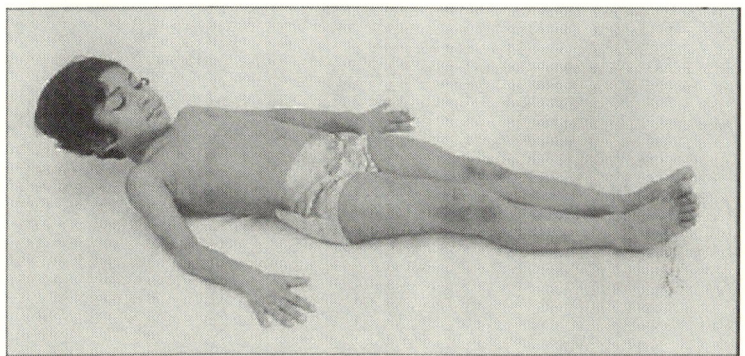

Figure 21 *Asana for the neck*

Lie down on your back. Put your feet together and arms at a little distance from your body. Raise your neck slowly until you can see your heels (Fig. 21).

Stay in this position as long as you can comfortably. Do not put pressure on your hands and elbows. The neck should be raised with its own force and shoulders will rise slightly with it. Bring down your neck slowly. Repeat this a few times with short intervals. If you cannot raise your neck high enough to be able to look at your heels, do not get discouraged. It is only a matter of repeated practice.

The second asana for the neck provides a counter movement to the above and consists of bending the neck backwards. Stand straight with your feet slightly apart. Raise both your arms upwards with the palms of the hands facing each other. Join the palms. Bring folded hands slowly downwards while simultaneously taking the neck backwards and inhaling. Bring your folded hands down to your forehead (Fig. 22). Reverse the whole process by slowly exhaling; that is, taking your folded hands upwards and straightening the neck. There are three steps involved in the whole practice: 1) coming down with folded hands while bending the neck backwards and inhaling; 2) the still position with folded hands on the forehead and withheld breath; 3) taking the hands up, straightening the neck and exhaling at the same time. Do all the movements while exhaling and inhaling very slowly and smoothly. If the air is taken too quickly and too much, it will gush out too fast and you will not be able to do this asana. The interval of withholding the breath will increase also with various practices of *pranayama* which is our next subject of discussion.

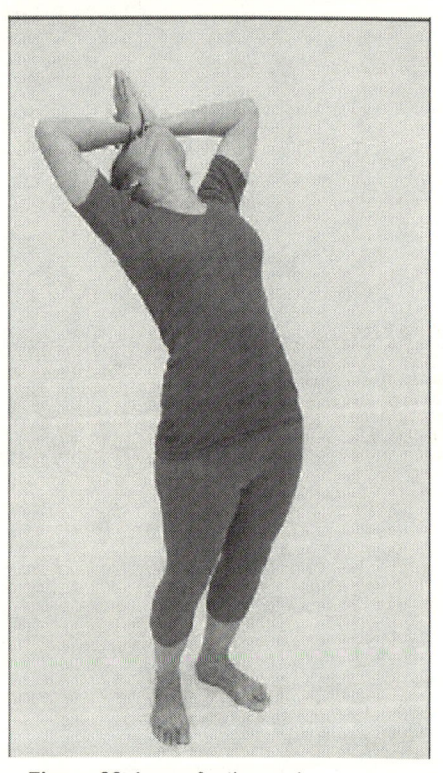

Figure 22 *Asana for the neck*

Possible difficulties: Some people have problems with bringing their folded hands up to their forehead. The reason for this is a slightly curved upper part of the vertebral column. The lifted arms are also not straight for these persons. This problem and its cure are discussed in the later part of the book (see Week VIII, A). Children cannot do this asana because their head is proportionately bigger.

Benefits: These two asanas provide exercise not only to the neck vertebrae and muscles, but also to the thorax region and to the upper back muscles, shoulders and arms. The second asana is also very good for the throat and the bronchial tube. In case of any throat and larynx infection, this asana might trigger a cough in the process of bending backwards.

Caution: People who have problems with their cervical vertebrae may not do these asanas. They are advised to cure these problems with the special asanas for the backbone (see Week IV, B).

E. *Pranayama*

Pranayama is the fourth of the eight fold yogic practices described by Patanjali (see Table 1). The literal meaning of *pranayama* is the expansion of vitality or vital energy. *Prana* is the vital energy which pervades everything, thus also the air we breathe in. To put it in simple words, *pranayama* involves the progressive deceleration of the respiratory rhythm achieved by prolonging inhalation and exhalation and increasing the central pause holding the breath. The latter involves two different steps; one is to hold the air inside the lungs and the other is to hold the lungs without air. *Pranayama* controls, regulates and balances the vital energy in the body and helps in attaining a thought free mind for the purpose of yoga.

I have already described some preparatory practices for *pranayama* in the previous chapter and now we will go into the technical details of this practice. *Pranayama* is done by regulating and controlling the physical breath. This latter involves three steps: 1. *puraka* is the process of taking air into the lungs; 2. *rechaka* is the process of letting the air out of the lungs; and 3. *kumbhaka* is holding the air inside the lungs (*antrik kumbhaka* or holding the lungs without air (*bahya kurnbhaka*).

The practice of Pranayama: There are many different practices of *pranayama* described in the yogic literature. We will take up some of them during the course of this book.

Sit down comfortably. See that your back and shoulders are straight and you are not tense. Close your eyes and bring your attention to the process of breathing. Slowly inhale the air until your lungs are filled (*puraka*). This process will expand your chest. When inhalation is complete, close both your nostrils with the help of your thumb and ring finger in order to hold the air inside the lungs (*antrik kumbhaka*). Simultaneously, release tension from your shoulders and back as these latter are under pressure due to the process of inhaling. Remove your fingers from your nostrils and let out the air slowly and smoothly (*rechaka*). Hold the nostrils once again to hold the lungs without air (*bahya kumbhaka*). In the beginning, do this practice only with single breaths, i.e., inhaling, holding with air, exhaling and holding without air. After these four steps, take a pause with normal breathing. When you acquire a slow and steady process of taking the air in and out and you feel that you are adept in *antrik kumbhaka* (holding the air inside the lungs), then follow the exhaling by *bahya kumbhaka*. After letting the air out from the lungs (*rechaka*), close your nostrils again as has been described before and hold the lungs for 1 to 2 seconds without air. Remove your fingers and begin to inhale slowly (*puraka*). Do not force yourself to do *rechaka*, *puraka* and *kumbhaka* for a longer time. The time should be gradually increased. Your attention should be completely on the process of *pranayama*. In the beginning, this practice should not be done for more than 5 to 6 minutes.

Benefits: The *pranayama* practices help in harmonizing the body and the mind. They strengthen the nervous system, increase memory and bring calmness and longevity. They are indispensable for other yogic practices. The specific therapeutic applications of some *pranayama* practices are described along with their description in the later part of the book.

Caution: The *pranayama* practices should not be done in stuffy rooms where the air is stale. It is better to do these practices in the open air or with at least an open window.

THIRD WEEK

A. Reflections on the Previous Learning

I hope that by now you have assimilated the three important facts about the yogic practices:

    a.   The movements should be very slow and smooth, i.e., they should not be in a "stop and go" or jerky manner.

    b.   Breathing should be harmonized with the movements and should also be smooth and slow.

    c.   Concentration should also be on the parts involved in that particular practice.

It should also be evident by now that the yogic practices involve internal as well as external parts of the body and our mind. If you do not feel comfortable with the movements and breathing and feel that you are unable to concentrate, I would suggest that you continue with the programme of the previous two weeks and do it regularly. Repeated practice lends the mind stability and gives the body an accompanied flexibility. You will slowly begin to realize that as the stiffness of the body goes away, the stiffness of the mind lessens too. After this realization, one of my students once asked me, "What relaxes first, the body or the mind?" I was unable to answer this question. The body and the mind relax spontaneously and it is difficult to separate them in order to arrive at such analysis.

B. *Vakshasana* or the Asana for Thorax

Lie down on your stomach with your arms bent on both sides and palms down on the floor. Your hands should be nearly at the level of your chin. Your chin should be down on the floor. Raise your head by gradually inhaling. Take your head as far back as you can without lifting up the elbows from the floor (Fig. 23). The pressure is on the forearms and the elbows.

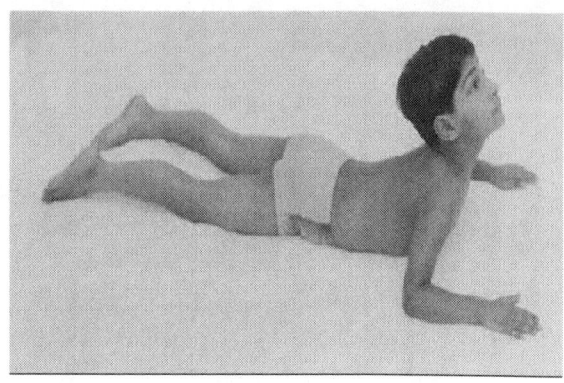

Figure 23 *Vakshasana*

Hold the air inside your lungs while in this position. Bring down your head by co-ordinated exhaling. Once your head is down, give yourself a rest of 3 to 4 breaths before repeating the practice. Repeat 8 to 10 times, concentrating always on the movement and harmonizing the breathing with it. Some of you may have to cough a little or clear the throat while doing this asana. But after doing it several times the blockaded in the thoracic area go away.

Benefits: This asana is very good for the throat and chest. It energizes the larynx and is useful for those who have to speak continuously for long hours. It also exercises the lungs.

C. *Gomukhasana*—A Posture for Chest and Arms

Gomukha means the mouth of a cow. It is called so because

of the position of hands joined at the back look like the mouth of a cow. You will encounter variations of this asana with different, teachers and from different books as far as the sitting posture is concerned. Some teachers or books instruct one to sit in *vajrasana* (Fig. 52) for making this posture. I do not think that a sitting posture is that important as this asana is principally concerned with the hands, arms, shoulders and chest. You may even stand and do it (Fig. 25).

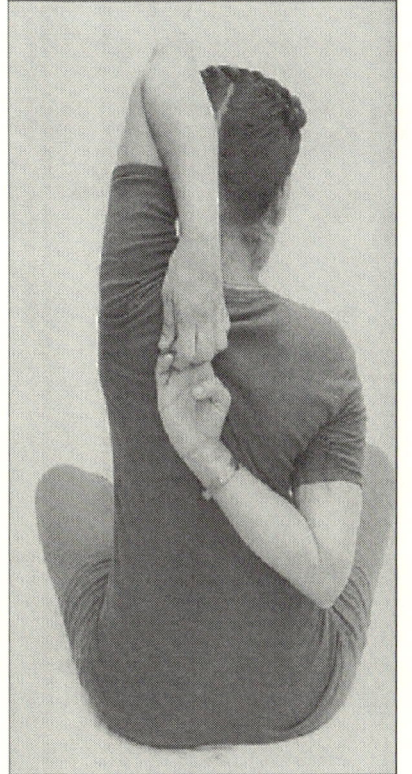

Figure 24 *Gomukha asana*

Sit in a comfortable posture, raise one hand and bring it behind your shoulder. Bend the other hand behind your back from the waist and join both hands together (Fig. 24). Breathing is automatically slowed down while sitting in this asana. Make this posture for a very short time in the beginning as it puts a great strain on the shoulder muscles and joints. You may gradually increase the time. Repeat 4 to 6 times by alternating the arms.

Possible difficulties: Many people realize that they cannot join the hands together. However, constant effort and regular practice of this asana and of other asanas, make this task possible. The muscles and joints of the body slowly acquire flexibility. Do not make the mistake of putting the palms of both hands towards the back like Abhinav has

81

done (see Fig. 25).

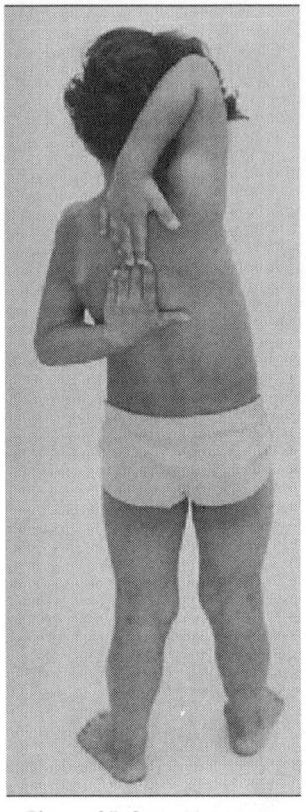

While doing this asana, one realises that there is a difference between the two sides of the body. A peculiarity about this asana is that for all of us (do not think that you are an exception), it is easier to join hands from one side than the other.

Benefits: This asana provides exercise to the shoulder joints, pectoral muscles and the muscles of the arms. It is very good for the chest muscles and is particularly recommended to women for strengthening the breast muscles and preventing the breasts from sagging. This asana gives a straight posture to the shoulders by providing equilibrium of energy in the left and right shoulders and arms.

Figure 25 *Gomukha asana*

This is needed because one shoulder is always lower than the other as most of us carry weights such as handbags etc., with our right hand or hang them on our right shoulder (vice versa for left-hand users).

D. Yogabhyasa for the Face Muscles

In the programme of last week, we have already had *yogabhyasa* where face muscles were actively involved (see Week II, B and C). The face musculature is very complicated and various muscles extend in different directions. The following practice provides an additional exercise to these muscles.

Sit down in a relaxed posture. Fill your mouth with air, close your lips and press the air in your mouth on both sides in order to inflate the cheeks with the air pressure. Move this air upwards to inflate the portion above the upper lip. After a few seconds, move the air downwards to inflate the portion below the lower lip (Fig. 26). Rest for a few breaths and fill the mouth with air again. This time push the air upwards and downwards and sideways quickly. Also move the air inwards (by slightly sucking it in) and outwards (by bringing it in the mouth again). This will produce some sound.

Benefits: This practice increases the blood flow in the face muscles and invigorates the face. It strengthens the face muscles and skin and prevents wrinkling.

Suggestions: If you find it difficult to do this exercise with the air in your mouth, you may do it with water. It is recommended to do this practice with water after meals and after having eaten sweet stuff for the care of gums and teeth. The water along with air forms a jet in the mouth and cleans the spaces between the teeth and the gums. One must direct this jet in different directions of the mouth with muscular pressure.

E. Chakshu Yoga (Yogabhyasa for the Eyes)

The organ of sight has a very complex anatomy. The eyelids and eyeballs move all the time. The yogic practices for the eyes involve controlling those reflex movements and doing some other movements consciously. Following are some yogic practices for the eyes.

1. Sit down in a convenient posture. Look straight ahead and slowly move your eyeballs upwards (Fig. 27). Your head should stay still and the forehead

83

should be smooth. Only your eyeballs should move. You will be able to see a part of your eyebrows by this practice. Bring the eyeballs in the centre again, give a little pause and now move them downwards so that you can look at your cheeks and nose (Fig. 28). Bring your eyeballs to the centre again and then move them to the extreme left and then to the extreme right (Figs. 29, 30). Repeat all four practices 5 to 10 times.

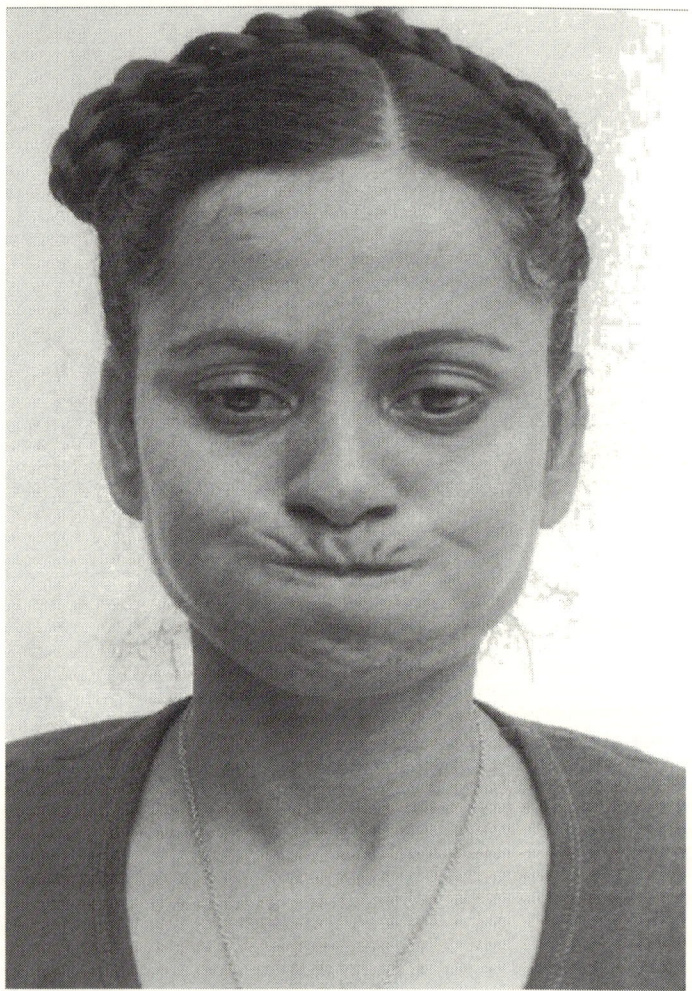

Figure 26 *Yoga for face muscles*

84

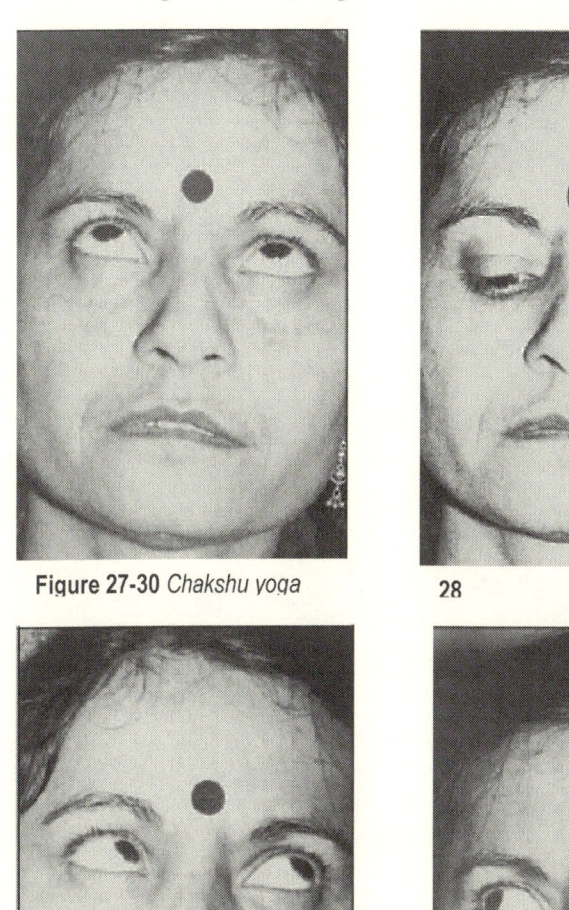

Figure 27-30 *Chakshu yoga*   28

29   30

2. This practice involves the incorporation of all the four
   above described exercises. It is done by making
   circular movements with the eyeballs. Figs. 27 to 30
   show one round of such movement. Give a small pause

after each circular movement and repeat 5 to 10 times or according to your feeling and capacity. Do not do these practices with the eyeballs if you feel tired, have a headache or after sitting in a moving vehicle for a long time.

3. This practice is done to provide energy to the eyes by looking at the sun. Since direct sunlight is harmful and even dangerous for the eyes, this practice is done by looking at the sun by various indirect ways.

   • Take two leaves, bring them close to your eyes and look at the sun through them. Concentrate your thoughts on the power of the sun and think of it as the source of life on our planet. Do not stare, just look normally. Staring is, in fact, harmful for the eyes.

   • The second exercise in this direction is to face the sun with closed eyes and to move the neck sideways in order to expose all parts of the eyes to the sun. One can look directly at the rising or the setting sun.

   • The third exercise is to look at the sun's reflection in water. A regular practice of this helps strengthen the eyesight.

Benefits: These yogic exercises remove tension and exhaustion from the eyes. They exercise the eye muscles and strengthen the nerves. They help improve the vision.

FOURTH WEEK

A. Reflection on the Previous Learning

As you progress with learning yogic practices, they become more and more comprehensive and involve your entire body. They also demand more of your concentration to coordinate the various movements with the breathing process. Thus, the difficulty is not only the inability of the body to twist and turn in a required way but also to stop background thought process and to concentrate in obtaining a balanced posture. One cannot make a posture steady without constant attention. The more one concentrates, the easier it becomes to overcome physical difficulties.

Pranayama is one way to obtain a thought-free mind. Besides, I have also invented some simple exercises to calm down the excitement of the mind and to stop the mind from wandering. These exercises prove to be very useful if one feels disturbed by something or is in a state of hyper-excitability and feels that one does not have control on one's thoughts anymore. Try the following simple exercises to quieten your mind.

The first exercise simply consists of taking some steps but in a special way. The left foot proceeds, then the right, then the left again and then the right. Now immediately proceed with the right foot and continue as before. In other words, walk normally four steps and then suddenly alternate the foot. You will realize that it is impossible to do this exercise without your entire attention.

The second exercise is inspired from the steps of a classical Indian dance, *Kathak*. It consists of tapping the feet on the floor softly as follows: left, right, left, right and then immediately right, left, right and left. It goes in this order: 1,2,3,4;4,3,2,1;1,2,3,4, and so on. In the beginning the speed will be rather slow and as soon as you will try to increase the speed, you will make a mistake in alternating the feet. It takes a lot of practice to do these movements fast and correct. Tapping should be done softly otherwise you might hurt your knees.

These exercises help stop the chain of thoughts in the mind and the thinking process gets involved in the physical activity. Yogic practices are always done with complete concentration of the mind.

B. *Prishthavanshasanas*— Backbone postures

These six asanas are probably the most important of the whole yogic practices described in this book as far as their therapeutic application is concerned. In our modern times, there are very few people who do not have one problem or another with their back. Many people suffer from various ailments connected to the cervical vertebrae, others have a curve in the thoracic vertebrae and a large number of desk workers have pain in the lower part of their back. These six asanas for the backbone cure any of these problems provided they are done regularly and other precautions are also taken for the care of the back. People who have problems with their back should never sleep in soft beds. They should get rid of excess weight and paunch. They should sit straight and should not bend their shoulders. Long sitting sessions should be interrupted with walks or just getting up and moving around.

The principal movements are the same in all the six asanas. The postures vary slightly for providing exercise to different parts of the backbone and the back muscles. The first three asanas are done lying on the back whereas the other three are done lying on the stomach.

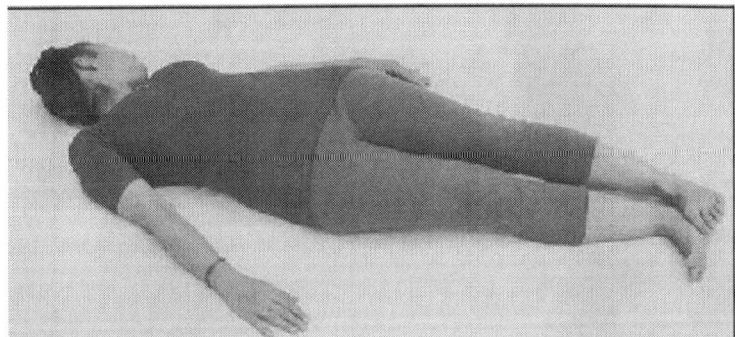

Figure 31 *Prishthavashasana*

1. Lie down on your back with hands apart from the body (about 30 centimetres) and both feet together.

Take some deep breaths and relax completely. After lying still for about 30 seconds, begin to turn your joined feet in one direction and your head in the opposite direction to the feet while slowly inhaling.

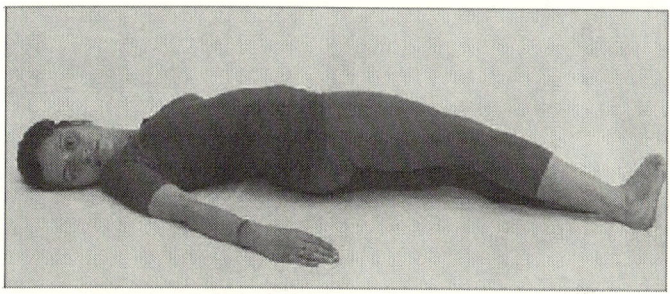

Figure 32 *Prishthavashasana*

When you have reached the farthest you can with both your feet and your head, relax your body from the effort of this movement while holding your breath (Fig. 31). Reverse this process slowly while exhaling and come back to the original straight position. Give yourself rest for a few breaths and repeat the same in the opposite direction (Fig. 32). Do the complete asana 10 to 15 times. Take care that you do not stretch your head too far out. The head should be straight and when in a turn position, it should be in the direction of your shoulder.

2. For the second asana, lie down the same way as above. Put one foot over the other (Fig. 33). Now slowly turn the feet in one direction and the head in the other while inhaling with the rhythm of the movement. When the movement is complete, let your body relax from the effort of the movement while the breath is withheld in this position (Fig. 34). Now slowly come back to the straight position while exhaling at the same rate as the pace of the movement. Pause for a few breaths before doing the same for the opposite direction (Fig. 35). When both the sides are done, bring the upper foot down and

repeat the asana by alternating the feet. Repeat 10 to 15 times.

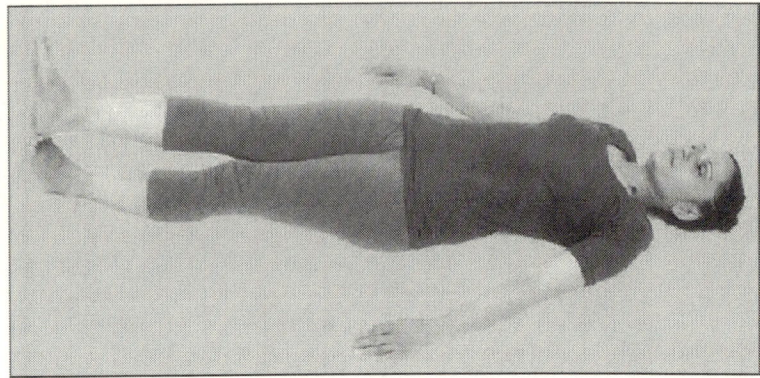

Figure 33 *Prishthavashasana*

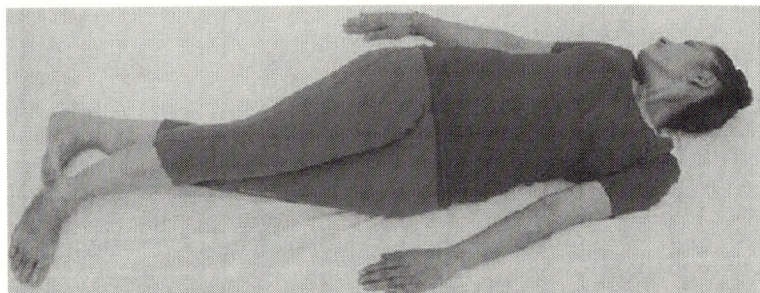

Figure 34 *Prishthavashasana*

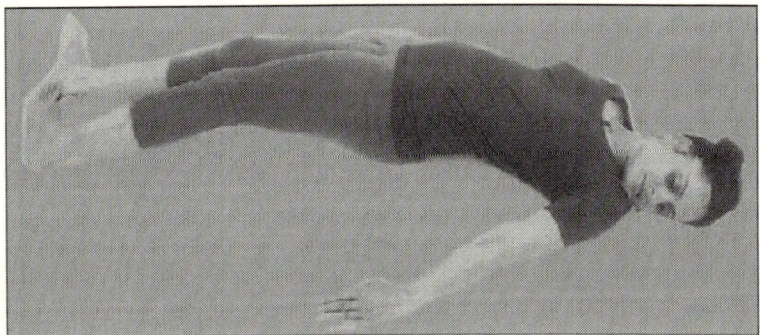

Figure 35 *Prishthavashasana*

3. The third asana in this series comprises of doing the same movements as in the above-described two asanas but with bent legs (Fig. 36). Turn the folded

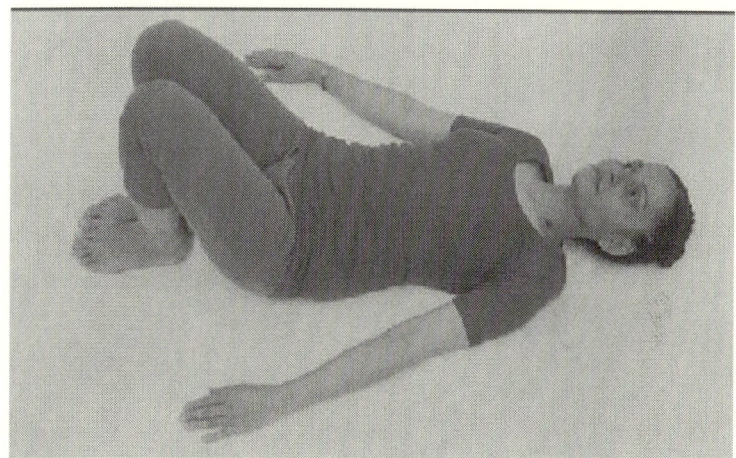

Figure 36 *Prishthavashasana*

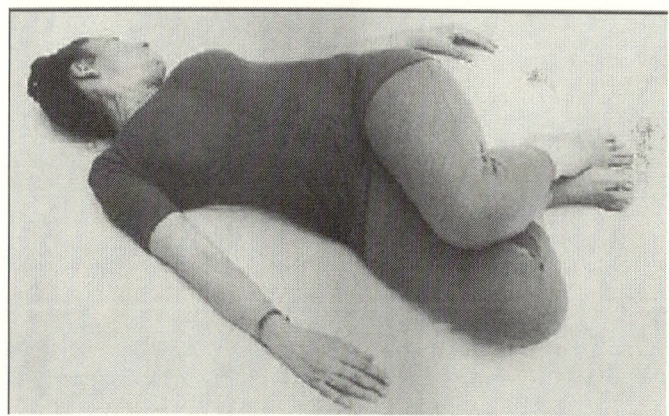

Figure 37 *Prishthavashasana*

legs in one direction and the head in the opposite direction while inhaling slowly and smoothly. Once the side of your leg touches the floor and the head is turned in the opposite direction, relax and hold the breath (Fig. 37). Release slowly the breath while coming back gradually to the straight position. Take a pause of a few breaths and repeat the same for the opposite direction (Fig. 38). Do this asana also 10 to 15 times.

4. The next three asanas in this series (4-6) are essentially the same as the first three but here the movements are done while lying on your stomach. While lying on the ventral side of the body, the head and the feet (or the leg) movements cannot be done in the opposite direction, thus they are done in the same direction.

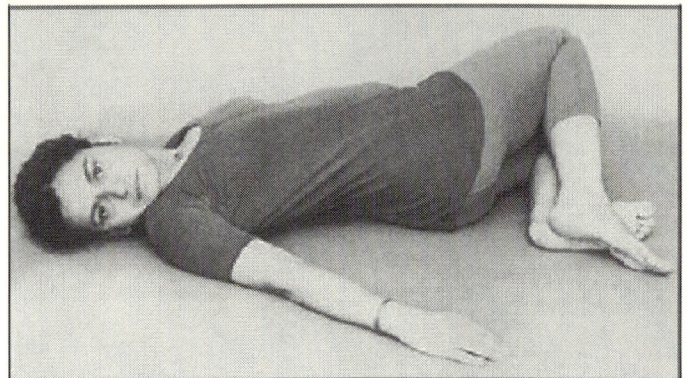

Figure 38 *Prishthavashasana*

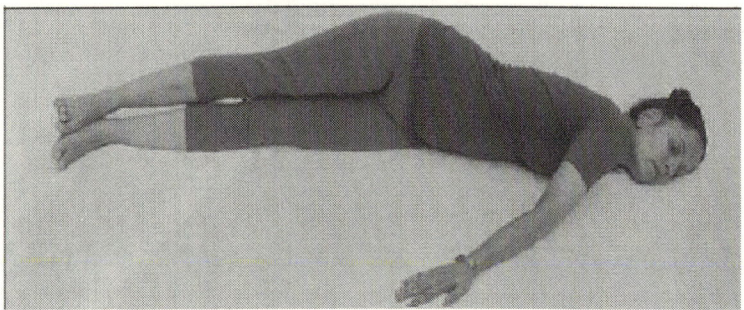

Figure 39 *Prishthavashasana*

Lie down on your stomach. Your chin should touch the floor and your feet should be together. Turn the joined feet and head simultaneously in the same direction while inhaling. Both your arms should stay straight, your cheek will touch the floor and your body weight will be on one side (Fig. 39). Relax and hold your breath in this position. Slowly, release your breath while returning to the starting position. Repeat the same movement in the opposite direction (Fig. 40).

The next asana entails placing your feet one above the other

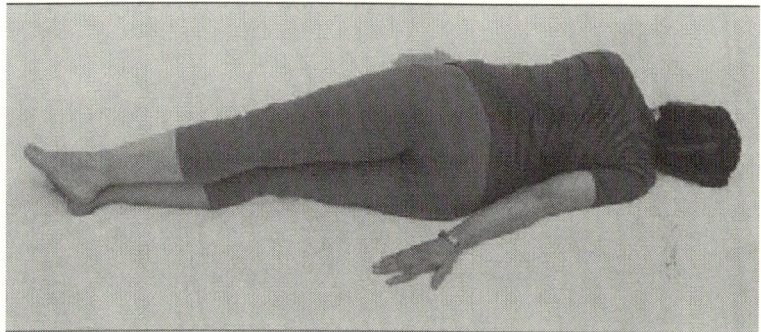

Figure 40 *Prishthavashasana*

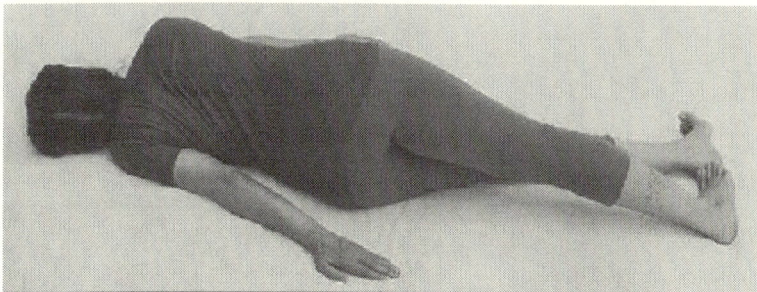

Figure 41 *Prishthavashasana*

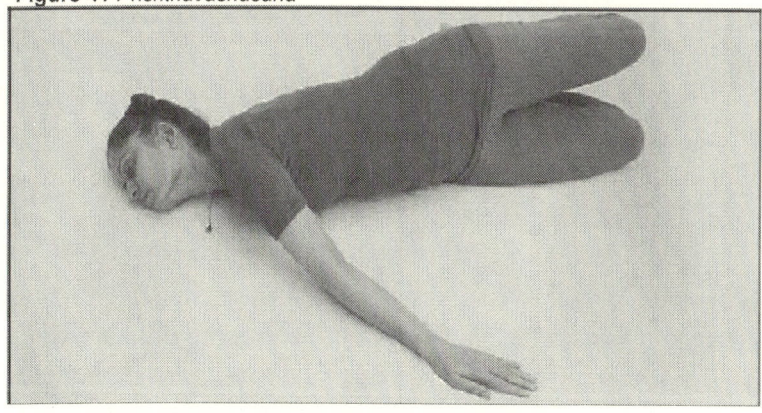

Figure 42 *Prishthavashasana*

as you did for the second asana of this series and doing the above-described movements (Fig. 41). Do not forget to alternate the position of the feet after you have completed turning in both directions. The sixth and the last asana of this series is done by bending back the legs and doing the same as above (Fig. 42). Repeat each of these asanas 10 to 15 times.

Possible difficulties: In the beginning, the difficulty is in coordinating the movements in two opposite directions and harmonising breathing with these two movements. You may first practice only the movements without paying attention to breathing. The second difficulty which most people face is that they inhale too quickly and take too much air into their lungs. The result is that they are unable to hold their breath while in the asana and the air gushes out with force. One should inhale very slowly so that the lungs are only half-full with air. This will help in holding the breath and in releasing it slowly during the process of recovery from the asana.

Benefits: The preliminary benefits of these asanas have already been stated. In addition, these asanas help to shed the fat around the waist and provide exercise to the large intestines.

B. Pranayama

In the first chapter, you have learnt about the subtle body within the human body which is represented by *nadis* or channels and is compared to the universe itself. The three principal *nadis* are *ida*, *pingala* and *sushumna*. *Ida* and *pingala* are on the left and right side of the backbone respectively and *sushumna* is in the middle. These three channels or *nadis* of the subtle body represent three gunas (moon channel) of the Cosmic Substance. *Ida*, also called *chandra nadi* influences the left part of the body and has *tamas guna* (the quality that resists motion). This *nadi* is cool in nature. *Pingala* or *surya nadi* (sun channel) has *rajas guna* (the quality that imparts motion). It provides heat and controls the right part of the body. The flow of *prana* into these two *nadis* is done by the left and right nostrils respectively. The *sushumna nadi* which is also called *shakti* or *sarasvati nadi* is in the centre of the *ida* and *pingala* and it is in this *nadi* that the *prana shakti* (the power of vital air) unites. It is neither hot nor cold and has *sattva guna* (the quality of virtue and balance).

To obtain a proper balance in the body, an equilibrium between *ida* and *pingala* is required. According to the Indian medical system, Ayurveda, besides the balance of the three energies of the body (vata, pitta and kapha), the balance of three *gunas* is also essential for health and harmony. In other words, we are attacked by a disease, when there is an imbalance between the energies of *ida* and *pingala*. The aim of the *pranayama* is to attain *sattva* by effecting a proper balance between *rajas* and *tamas* and that is done by bringing an equilibrium between *ida* and *pingala* which are opposite in nature.

Purification of *nadis* called *nadi shodhana* is practiced as a first step in *pranayama* for achieving a proper balance in the body. The basic technique is the same as described previously (see Week II, E) with the difference that for *nadi shodhana* the vital energy or *prana* is canalised through one nostril at a time. The first step of this practice is to clean *ida* and *pingala* individually and the second step is to canalise the vital force in a circle through both these *nadis* to create a balance of energy.

Sit in a comfortable posture. Close your right nostril with the thumb of your right hand and inhale slowly and smoothly till the lungs are filled with air. Now close also the left nostril with the ring finger of the same hand and hold the *prana* inside. The next step is to lift the ring finger from your left nostril and exhale slowly and smoothly. The right nostril should remain closed all the time during this practice. Do this practice 8 to 10 times. This purifies the *chandra nadi* or *ida*. Now do exactly the same with your right nostril to purify *surya nadi* or *pingala*. During this practice, your left nostril remains closed with the thumb of your left hand. Repeat as many times as the previous practice. For the second part of the *nadi shodhana* practice, inhale the vital energy or *prana* through your left nostril while your right nostril is closed with the thumb of your right hand. Close your left nostril also with the ring finger of the same hand. Then release the air from your right nostril while the left one is kept closed. Do *bahya kumbhaka* by closing both your nostrils and begin inhaling this time from your right nostril. In other words, you are circulating *prana* from *ida* to *pingala* and then from *pingala* to *ida*. In order not to get confused with the left and right sides, remember this: "in from left, holding in, out from right, holding out, in from right, holding in and so on". Repeat 8 to 10 times.

Benefits: The *nadi shodhana* practice strengthens the nerves and brings calmness. It enhances the capacity of concentration. People who are nervous and restless are specially advised to do this practice. It is also useful in getting rid of headaches which are due to nervous tension and is recommended to those suffering from migraines. Sometimes one gets pain in one side of the head or face due to a partial blocking of the nostril. This practice helps detect this and cures such pains. Minor nasal infections can be cured by doing this practice with the vapours of various oils as mentioned in Chapter 2.

D. Significance of "Om" and its Recitation

We have already discussed the syllable "OM" and the

meaning of this symbol according to the Yoga Sutras of Patanjali (see Fig. 2). "OM" symbolizes *Brahman* or the Universal Soul. This monosyllable is composed of three phonemes: A, U and a nasal M. It is considered the smallest *mantra*. The three phonemes of this syllable unite in themselves the existential multiplicity and its unity with the Absolute.

In the brief description of *Sankhya* in Chapter 1, it has already been said that the two fundamental realities of the universe are the *Purusha* and the *Prakriti*. The *Purusha* is the animating principle of the *Prakriti*. It is that which breathes life into matter. "OM" is the symbolic representation of the *Purusha*. In other words, "OM" is symbolic of Cosmic Consciousness. This consciousness is beyond the subjective consciousness of our inner world of thoughts, feelings and desires. It is beyond words and concepts and thus, is represented only by a monosyllable.

I have repeatedly talked about harmonizing breathing and the body movements. The recitation of "OM" is for the purpose of harmonizing our whole being with the universe. The recitation of "OM" is synchronized with breathing. Begin by repeating the word "OM" with each breath. Slowly increase the time of recitation by prolonging the sound AU and ending by a nasal "M". Take a deep breath each time and begin reciting very softly by slowly raising the pitch and again lowering it at the end while pronouncing "M". Repeat several times without a break. During recitation, the eyes should be closed and the symbol "OM" should be visualized at a point between the two eyes.

Benefits: With the chanting of "OM" begins the process of purification of the mind. It is a very personal experience for each one of you which is beyond words.

Note: For more details about OM, its recitation and benefits, please consult my book on AUM: The Eternal Energy.

FIFTH WEEK

A. General Discussion

At one time or the other in our lives, we go through an experience when we realize that despite all our efforts, we were unable to achieve something that we had so desperately wanted. Many times, we want to finish something in a limited period of time and we over-work for that. Despite fatigue and lack of energy, we do all to complete a piece of work. We proceed with strict planning and discipline. Yet, in spite of all our efforts, sometimes, we cannot achieve what we want to. We are prevented by a sudden illness or an accident or some similar mishap. These incidents in our lives should not be ignored. Rather, they should help to teach us a lesson. Probably, an obstruction happens because we bring ourselves to the point of exhaustion.

According to the philosophy of yoga, nothing happens without reason and the universe is a perfectly organized whole. Nothing stays forever. Decay, aging and death are the principles of existence. Only the Essence or the Absolute or the Universal Soul or Purusha is eternal. Existence, as we know it, comes to an end in its totality one day, and returns to the Cosmic Substance—Prakriti and the Essence of all beings is reabsorbed in to the Universal Soul—Purusha. Another cosmic cycle begins by the combination of Purusha and Prakriti. It is due to this fundamental philosophy of cosmic cycles that a wheel or a chakra has a symbolic significance and dharma is represented with a wheel with radiating beams[17]. On a smaller time scale, there is a cycle of birth and death—sansara. The points of energy in the subtle body are also represented by chakras.

---

[17] *The wheel or chakra that adorns the Indian National Flag also symbolizes dharma*

If we are obstructed and have hindrances or obstacles, like falling ill or other incidents of this sort then there must be a reason for it. A greater understanding of ourselves and of the system of this universe might help us to find the cause of negative happenings and help us to prevent them. Blaming happenings on coincidence is nothing but an acknowledgement of our ignorance. We bring ourselves to an extreme point of fatigue, exhaustion and nervousness when we become prey to accidental mistakes.

Stop yourself from getting confused, nervous and absentminded. Be completely involved in what you are doing and concentrate fully on your actions; the process of consciousness begins from here. Paying attention makes us aware and awareness is essential for consciousness. Take for example something very simple—a bad habit like biting your nails. When you bite your nails, a friend might say, "You are doing this again, stop it." You may say, "Yes, I know that I should not do this." Yes, you know that but you are not conscious of this bad habit. To gain consciousness about this bad habit of yours, hold a special session, 4 to 5 times a day of biting your nails. Sit down comfortably, take some deep breaths and start biting your nails. Repeat it a few times. If you do this practice regularly, after a few times, your fingers will no longer automatically move to your mouth in order to get bitten. You may try this method with any of the bad habits you want to get rid of.

B. *Bhujangasana* or the Serpent Posture

Lie down on your stomach with your chin on the floor. Bend your arms and put your hands on the floor nearly at the level of your chest. Now raise your head and chest slowly while inhaling. There will be pressure on your hands and your arms will straighten in this process. Bend as far back as you can (Fig. 43). Stay in this position for a few seconds and then slowly return to the starting position while exhaling. In this asana, very little air is inhaled during the process of bending backwards and that air is pushed back to

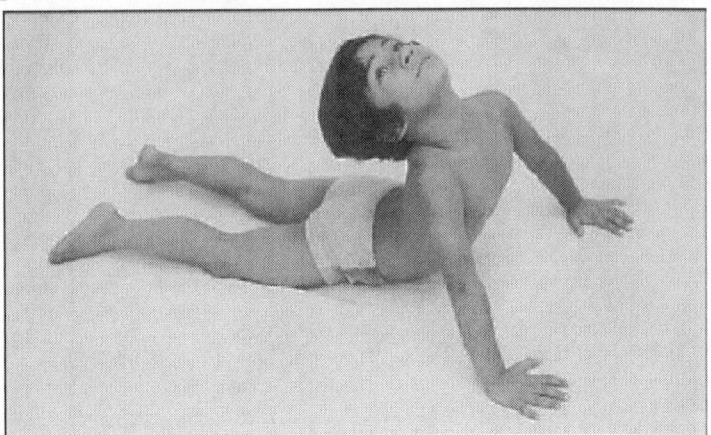

Figure 43 *Bhujangasana*

the farthest part of the lungs by this posture. The air is also released automatically during the recovery process from this posture. Repeat 8 to 10 times and allow an interval of a few breaths between each performance. For therapeutic application, gradually increase the frequency and do up to 20 times daily.

Possible difficulties: Do not get discouraged if you cannot go as far back as Abhinav (See Fig. 43). It is not advisable to suddenly bend too far back. You may get cramps not only in your chest or back muscles but also in your arms and shoulders.

Benefits: This asana strengthens the vertebral column and gives elasticity to the back. It is very good for the purification of the lungs and is specially recommended to those suffering from bronchitis, asthma, chronic cough or any other lung infection. This asana vitalizes the smooth muscles of the digestive tract. It helps to shed abdominal fat and prevents the abdominal muscles from getting loose with aging. It also makes the arms stronger.

C. *Padahastasana* or the Hand to Feet Posture

This asana is done standing and comprises of bringing down slowly the raised hands and touching the feet with them. (Figs. 44-46). Stand relaxed with feet slightly apart. Release tension from your body and straighten your shoulders and backbone. Concentrate on your body and its form in this erect position. Now slowly raise both your arms parallel to each other with palms facing forwards (Fig. 44). Once in this position, start bending forwards slowly while inhaling. During the process of bending, your head should stay parallel to your arms and you should bend from the lower part of your back. Your knees should not bend. Bend down as far as you can and touch your feet with your hands (Fig. 45). Either withhold the breath in this position or continue breathing at a low rate. This latter is done when one stays in this asana longer than a few seconds. Slowly recover from this position and come back to the standing posture. Repeat 5 to 7 times with short intervals.

Possible difficulties: There are two major difficulties in making this asana. Most people are not flexible enough to be able to touch their feet without bending their knees. One should go as far as one can but without bending the knees. Each time one should try to go slightly above the threshold. While bending, try to stretch yourself forwards from the lower part of your back and then lean down to touch your feet. Do not force yourself to achieve quick success otherwise you will have pain in the thigh and calf muscles. These muscles stretch tremendously during this posture. Wisdom lies in being slow and steady to achieve the goal. In spite of their flexible bodies, children have difficulty in doing this asana, as their arms are proportionately shorter (Fig. 46).

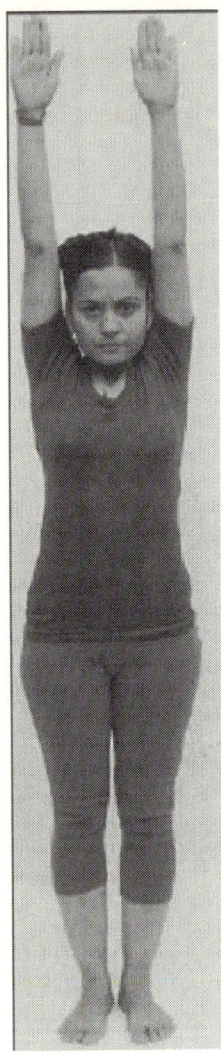

Figure 44
Padahastasana

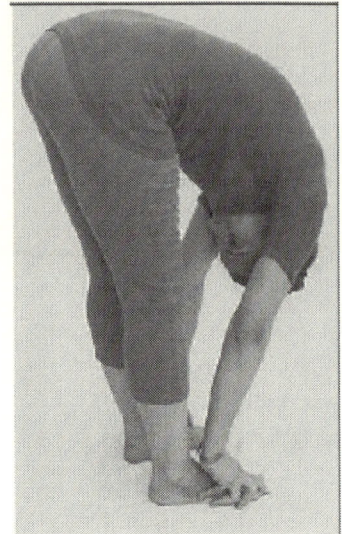

Figure 45 *Padahastasana*

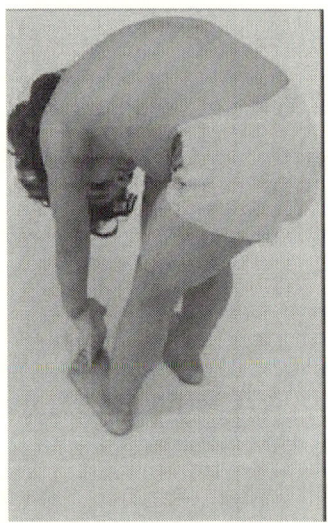

Figure 46 *Padahastasana*

Benefits: This asana is particularly good for the urinary system, uterus and for the secretion of seminal fluids. It helps to regulate the menstrual cycle and to get rid of

102

menstrual pains. It also cures constipation. This asana makes the backbone and spine strong and flexible and strengthens the thigh and calf muscles.

D. *Ardhachakrasana* or the Half-Wheel Posture

This asana provides a counter movement to the previous asana. As the name suggests, it consists of making a half wheel or *chakra* with your body. Stand straight in a relaxed posture as has been described before. Put the palms of your hands on your hips and slowly start bending backwards.

Go as far back as you can. Your hands on your hips will provide a support for bending backwards (Fig. 47). Stay for a few seconds in this position and slowly return to the

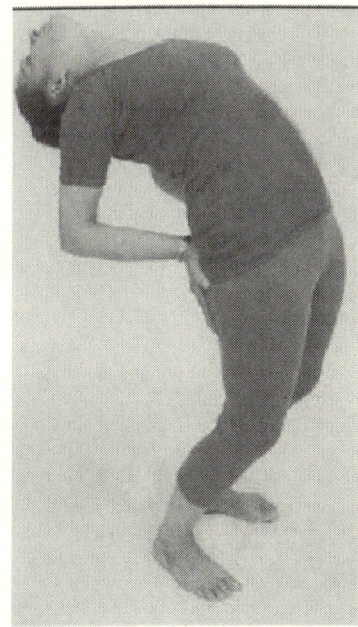

straight posture. Breathing is automatically regulated during this asana. During the first half of bending backward, there is an intake of a little quantity of air which is held inside during this asana. During the second half of this posture, this air is automatically released. Repeat 5 to 8 times with short pauses in between. Do not force yourself to bend too much. Remember that the success in yogic postures is achieved by perseverance and concentration and not by force.

Figure 47 *Ardhachakrasana*

Possible difficulties: Some people lose their balance while bending backwards. Keep your feet firmly on the floor to maintain a proper balance and do not bend too far back in the beginning. Some others may feel giddy in this posture or in other such postures that entail bending backwards. If this is the case then do not stay in this position. Just bend backwards and come forward immediately.

Benefits: During many of our daily activities, we bend forwards and this kind of backward movement provides a balance and redistributes the body's energy. This asana also promotes circulation of blood into the head and cures headaches. It is good for the spinal nerve and provides flexibility to the back. It cures backaches of muscular origin.

Caution: Those who have problems with their spine or vertebral discs should not do this asana. They are advised to concentrate first on the six backbone asanas to cure themselves.

E. Continuation of *Pranayama Kapalabhati*

Kapalabhati means to clean the head. Sit down in a comfortable position and inhale through both your nostrils till your lungs are full with air. During this process, concentrate on the *prana* or the vital energy you are taking inside you. Relax your shoulders and back once the process of inhaling is complete and start exhaling the air from your lungs with full force. Empty your lungs completely by forcing out the last remaining air from the deepest parts of your lungs. This process will retract your stomach, will put pressure on the lower part of your throat and will also take out the abdominal air. Repeat this practice by changing the passage of *prana* by alternating inhaling through oral and nasal passages. For example, inhale air through the nasal passage and take it out through the mouth and then inhale through the mouth and take it out through the nostrils.

Benefits: Your head will feel cool after this practice. *Kapalabhati pranayama* is very useful in obtaining a thought-free mind and it increases the power of concentration. It cleans the lungs and provides exercise to the stomach, larynx, trachea and bronchial tubes.

SIXTH WEEK

A. *Dhanurasana* or the Bow Posture

This asana consists of making the shape of a bow with the body (Fig. 48). Lie down on your stomach. Relax completely and think about the form of your body. Bend your legs so that your ankles will either touch or will be quite close to your hips. Now lift up your arms and reach backwards to hold your ankles. Tighten your grip on your ankles and lift your body from the floor by applying force from your hands and arms (Fig. 48). By doing this, your thighs and a part of your thoracic region will lift up. Abdominal region of your body will bear most of your weight. Breathing is automatically regulated as very little air can stay inside the lungs during this asana. The air is automatically thrown out when you return to the normal position. Stay in this asana for a few seconds. Repeat 5 to 7 times with an interval of 30 seconds each time. You may do *shavasana* after this asana in order to relax from the effort of this asana.

Possible difficulties: This asana requires the flexibility of the whole of your body. If you have been regularly doing the other yogic practices described until now, you will not find this asana difficult. Some people find it difficult to apply force from the hands when the arms are stretched backwards. Act as though you were lifting up something which is lying behind you. Some others have difficulty in reaching their ankles with their hands. You should make an effort to bring your ankles as much forwards as possible so that you may gain some space. This asana is difficult for children as their arms are proportionately smaller.

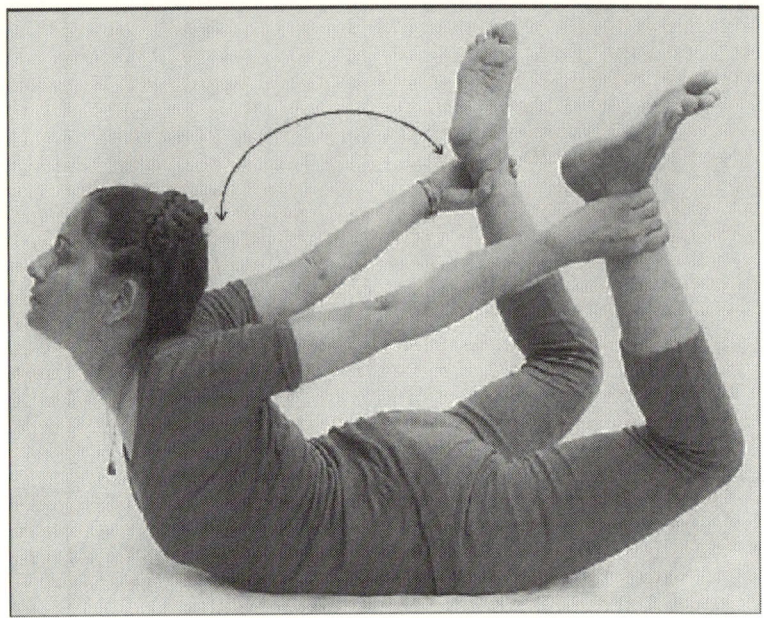

Figure 48 *Dhanurasana*

Benefits: This asana involves the whole of your body and thus gives exercise to all the internal organs, muscles and joints. It helps to shed off fat. This asana circulates the body's energy, thus, providing an equilibrium.

Caution: Those who have trouble with their spine or discs should not do this asana.

B. *Khagasana* or the Bird Posture

Khagasana is an extension of *dhanurasana*. It comprises in rocking with that part of your body which touches the floor when you are in *dhanurasana* (Fig. 48, arrows). You should rock forwards and backwards. Repeat the movement 4 to 6 times according to your capacity. Repeat this asana a few times with short intervals in between.

Benefits: This asana provides further impetus for circulating the body's energy and provides an equilibrium. The other benefits are the same as for the previous asana.

C. *Janusandhiasanas* or the Postures for the Knees

Our knees are very fragile and are easily injured. A lack of exercise makes them still more fragile and the result is that many people have problems with their knee joints. Following are some asanas to strengthen the knees.

1. Stand straight and loosen yourself. Make sure that your shoulders are not tense and your back is straight. Now bend one of your legs, bend slightly down to hold your foot with both your hands and pull it up in such a way that the sole of the foot is upwards (Fig. 49). The knee of the bent leg should not extend out too much. Try and make your body straight. Stay in this asana only for a few seconds in the beginning, slowly adapt your knee to this position and increase the time. Repeat 4 to 6 times with each leg. While in this posture, concentrate your thoughts on your knees. Your breathing will automatically slow down while you are in this asana. Force from your arms and hands is required to make this posture.

2. Stand in a similar way as described above. Bend one leg backwards. Bring both hands to your back, hold your bent leg by the ankle and pull it up slightly so that both your thighs are parallel (Fig. 50).

   Repeat 4 to 6 times for each leg by alternating the legs every time. To begin with, stay in his posture for a few seconds only and then gradually increase the time.

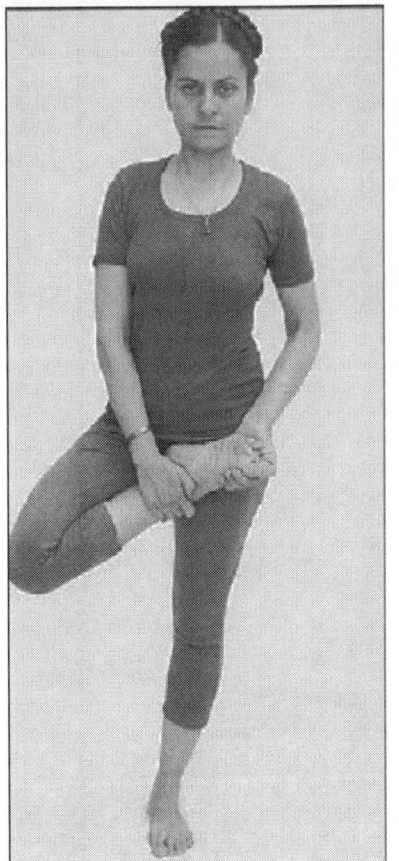

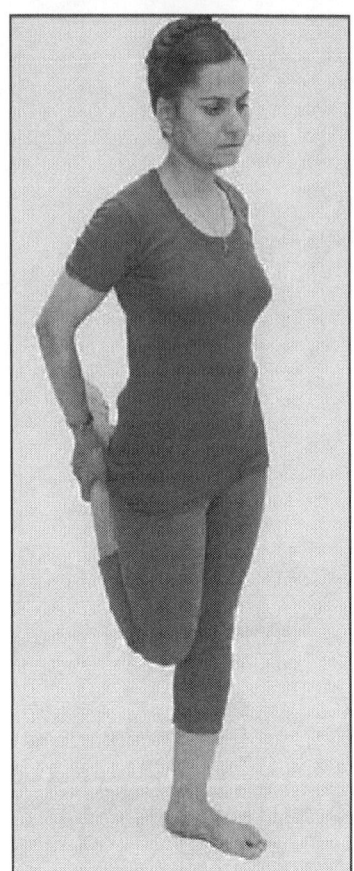

Figure 49 *Janusandhiasana*   **Figure 50** *Janusandhiasana*

3. The third and the last asana of this series is done by
   lifting one leg and putting the sole of the foot of this
   leg on the knee of the other leg (Fig. 51). The lifted
   leg should not extend forwards. Make an effort to
   pull it back and bring it to the level of the rest of the
   body. Repeat 4 to 6 times for each leg, alternating
   the legs every time. Increase the duration of the
   asana gradually.

Benefits: These asanas strengthen the knees and
prepare them for other more complex asanas. They are
also good as preparatory exercises for skiers.

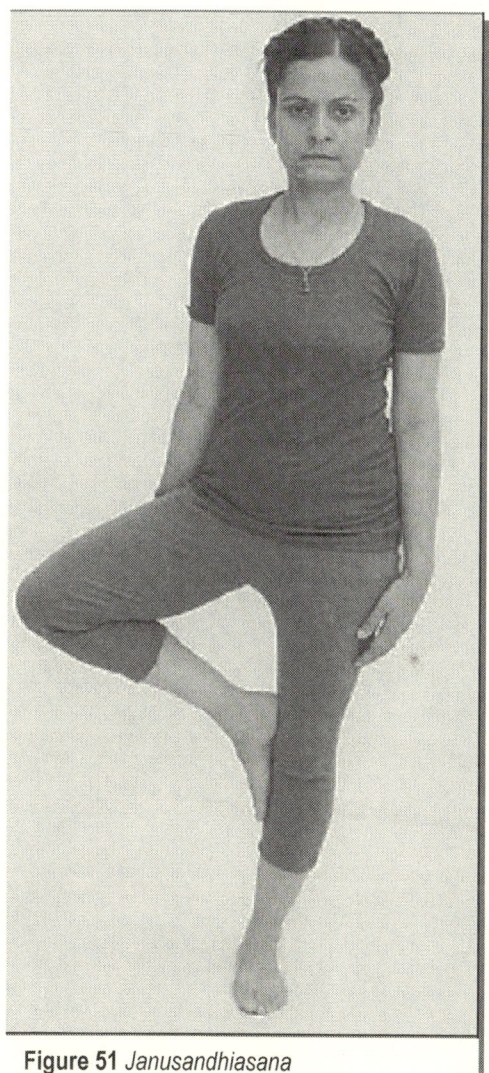

Figure 51 *Janusandhiasana*

Caution: Do not force yourself into fast success in making these postures as you may hurt your knees in this process. Be very indulgent and proceed gradually.

D. *Vajrasana* or the Rock Posture

Little Gayatri is sitting very comfortably in *vajrasana* (Fig. 52). This is one of the most difficult asanas for Western adults whereas children in the West often sit like this. The flexibility of the knees and the legs is lost as one grows up because it is not customary in the West to sit on the floor with bent legs. However, regular practice of the knee asanas will be helpful for making this posture. For those, who cannot do this asana and the other asanas related to it, an alternative is given (see Week VII, C).

Start by sitting on your heels. Then slowly move your legs (from the knees downwards) sideways, until your bottom is resting on the floor. Put your hands on your knees (Fig. 52). Sit in this asana for a brief period in the beginning in order not to overstrain the ankles, knees and pelvic joints. Once you have mastered sitting in this asana, you may use it for doing *pranayama* practices, recitation of 'OM' and other concentration practices. This asana can also be used simply as a sitting posture to make the body strong and stable, thus the name *vajra* or rock asana.

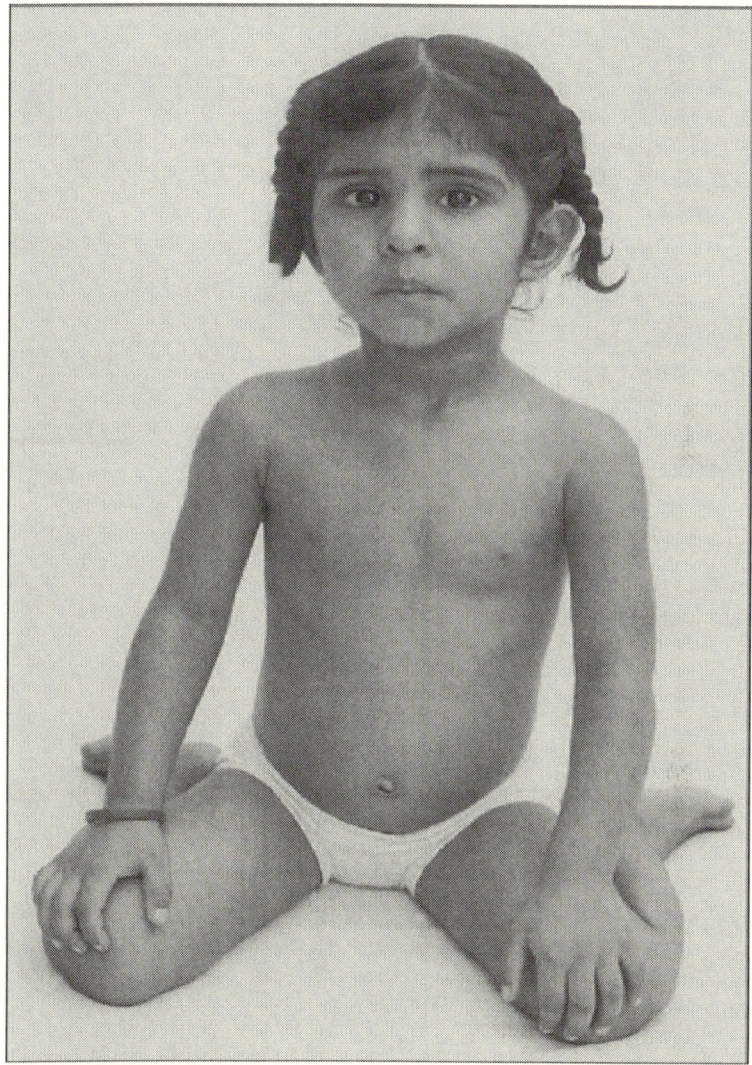

Figure 52 *Vajrasana*

Possible difficulties: The difficulty of sitting in this asana is due to a lack of flexibility in the knees, ankles and pelvic joints. Some people have problems in touching the floor with their hips due to stiff pelvic joints. Try each time for a few seconds in order to make the joints gradually flexible.

111

Obtaining a steady posture may take six months to one year with regular practice. Women find it easier to make this posture as compared to men.

Benefits: As said above, this asana makes the body strong and stable. It gives an erect posture to the spine and the shoulders. It also results in a harmonious blood flow in the body, thus, can prevent arteriosclerosis. This asana is especially good for people suffering from haemorrhoids (piles).

This asana can be practiced even after having eaten. It ensures good digestion. This asana also strengthens the leg muscles.

Caution: Do not force yourself; you may hurt your ankles, knees or pelvic joints. Do not sit in this asana longer than your capacity and only very gradually increase the time.

E. Pranayama

This week's programme of *Pranayama* comprises of doing the *nadishodhana* practice as has been described in the programme of the last week (see Week IV, C) but by directing the *prana* upwards. Begin this practice from your left nostril just as you did earlier but this time by directing the *prana* to the left side of your head. Concentrate fully to guide the *prana shakti* or vital power. After the *antrik kumbhaka*, slowly do *rechaka*, from your right nostril while the left remains closed with the ring finger of the right hand. Do the rest of the practice in the same way as before except that in this case the *prana* should be directed to the head and is circulated there.

Benefits: This practice is for the purification of the brain and strengthens the nervous system. It helps one to stay calm and increases the concentration power.

Finish the session with the recitation of "OM". This time, go into the details of the form of the figure "OM". As soon as you commence with the sound, bring your thoughts to the upper part of the figure and visualize the whole form of "OM" in your mind while simultaneously chanting. When you come to the nasal 'M', think of the half moon and the point in it in the figure "OM". This practice will help enhance your concentration and help your mind to relate the form to the sound.

SEVENTH WEEK

A. *Shashankasana* or the Moon Posture

Begin this asana by sitting in *vajrasana*, (see Week VI, D, Fig. 52). Once you are comfortably sitting in *vajrasana*,

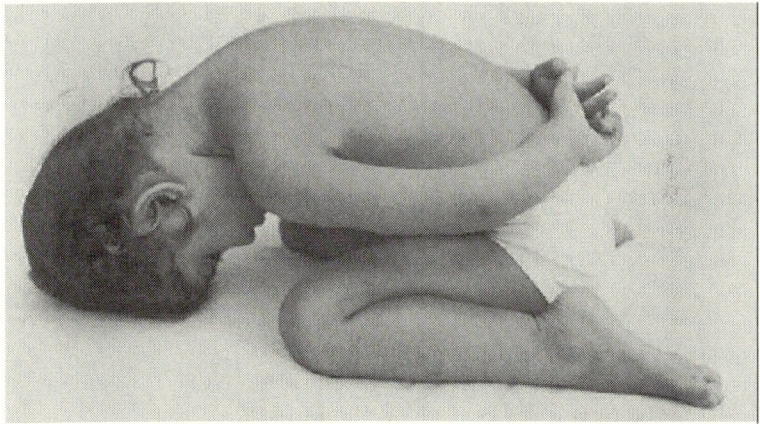

Figure 53 *Shashankasana*

move your hands to your back and hold them together. Now slowly begin to bend forward until your head touches the floor. Try to keep your hips as close to the floor as possible (Fig. 53). While bending, most of the air will be squeezed out from your lungs and when you are in this posture, breathing continues at a very low rate. In the beginning, make this asana only for a few seconds and repeat it after short pauses. Gradually increase the time, until you are able to stay in this posture up to one minute or more.

Benefits: This is a prophylactic asana against diabetes. It also provides exercise to all abdominal organs. It increases the blood flow to the face, forehead and top of the head and brings a glow to the face. It helps cure headaches of nervous origin.

B. *Suptavajrasana* or the Supine-Rock Posture

This asana also begins by sitting in *vajrasana* and consists

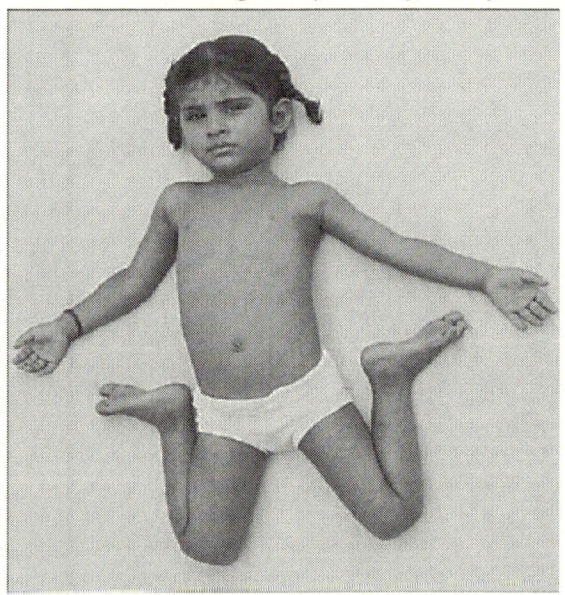

Figure 54 *Suptavairasana*

of lying on your back while you are in *vajrasana* (Fig. 54). One needs a very flexible pelvic joint to do this asana. Sit in *vajrasana* and slowly recline by taking the support of your elbows. Gradually lie down flat on your back and stretch your arms out on both sides (Fig. 54). You will realize that the frontal muscles of the thighs are greatly stretched during this asana and there is a pressure on the pelvic joint. Let yourself completely loose after making this posture. Stay in this asana as long as you can comfortably and gradually increase the time by a few seconds every session. In the beginning, you may repeat this asana by taking short pauses until you acquire a steady posture.

Benefits: This asana makes the ankle, knee and pelvic joints flexible and energizes the nerves and muscles of the legs, specially the front muscles of the thighs. It provides exercise to the hip muscles and enhances blood circulation in this region. Complementing *shashankasana*, this asana enhances blood circulation in the back of the head. This asana, accompanied by the raised leg asanas previously described (see Week 1, D) are specially suggested to people suffering from sciatic pains.

Alternatives to *Vajrasana*, *Shashankasana* and *Suptavajrasana*

An alternative posture to *vajrasana* is made by sitting erect on your heels with knees slightly apart and hands on the thighs (Fig. 55). In the previously described *vajrasana*, your legs (from the knee down) are on the side of your thighs and your hips are on the floor. This automatically gives you an erect posture. In this asana, you have to pay attention that your back and shoulders are straight. Make *shashanka* and *suptavajrasana* from this alternative posture the same way as described earlier (Figs. 56, 57). You will realize that because your feet are under your hips, your back will not touch the floor in this version of the *suptavajrasana* (Fig. 57). There is an additional way of making this posture; that is by touching the floor with the top of your head (Fig. 58) instead with the back of it (Fig. 57). I personally find this latter very relaxing and refreshing for the head and the nerves.

115

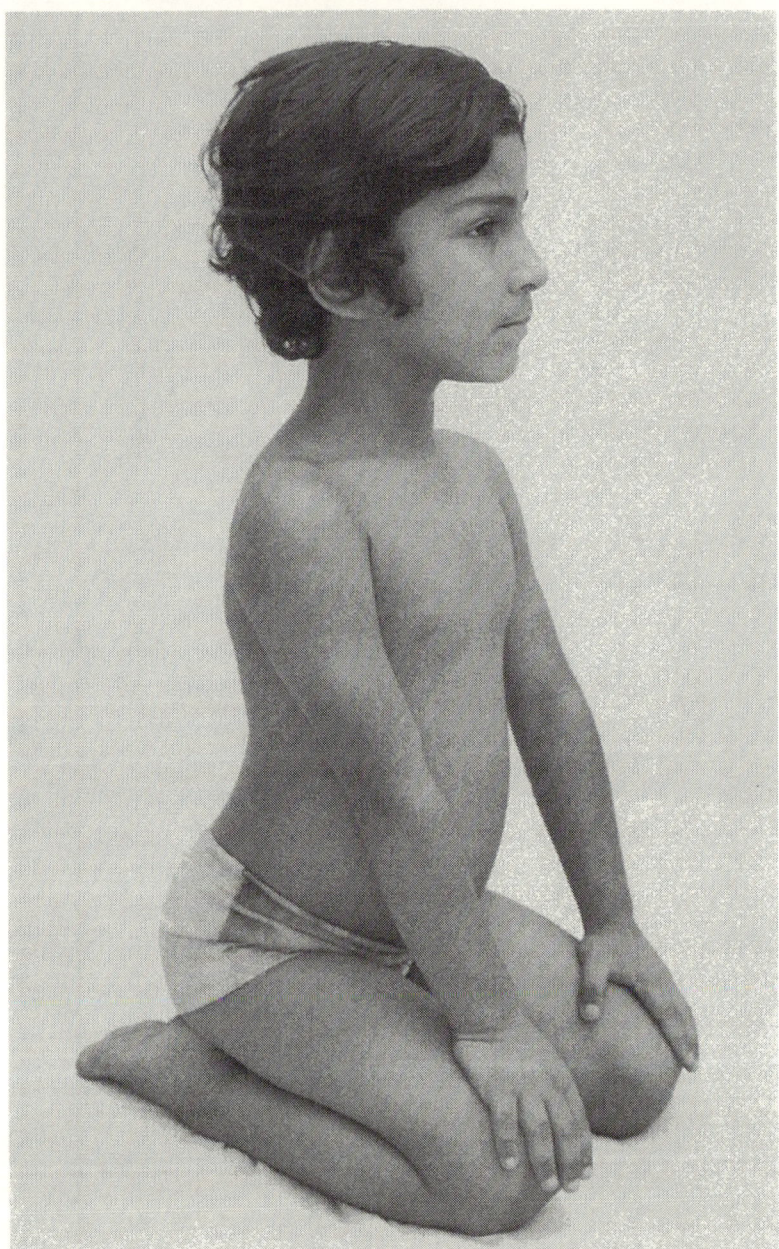

Figure 55 *Alternative to Vajarasana*

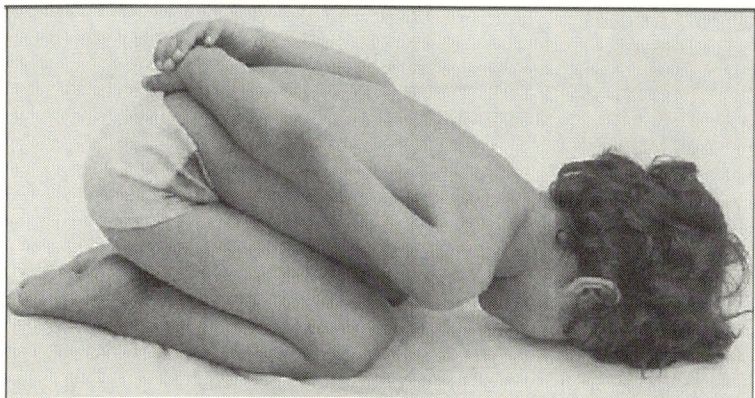

Figure 56 *Alternative to Shashankasana*

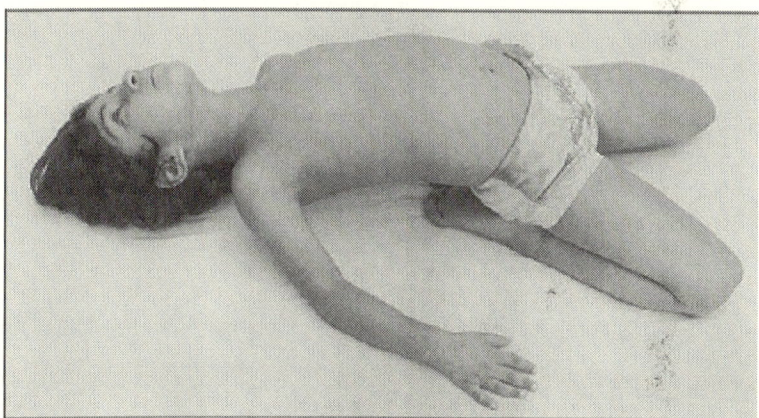

Figure 57 *Alternative to Suptavajarasana*

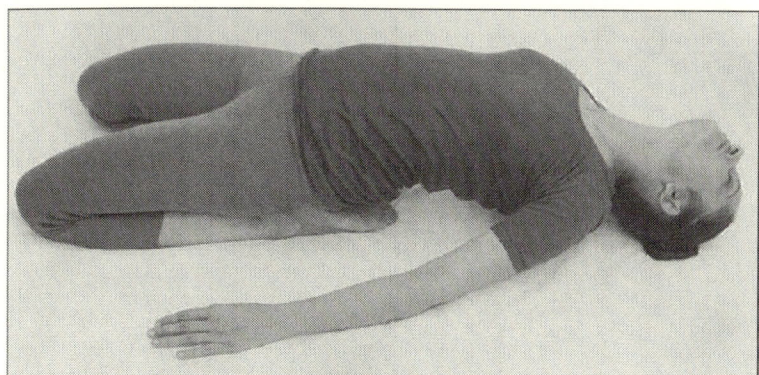

Figure 58 *Alternative to Suptavajarasana*

D. *Pranayama*

This week's programme of *pranayama* includes the revision of all the practices learnt until now and to learn to increase the time for *puraka*, *rechaka* and *kumbhakas*. The secret for increasing the time depends upon the following two factors: 1) your complete concentration on the *prana* you are taking in; and 2) a state of complete relaxation of the body. Your thought process and *prana* should be completely in rhythm with each other, your eyes should be closed and your ears should only hear the sound produced by the passage of vital air. Your senses should be closed to anything else outside the micro-cosmos of your body which is in connection with the macro-cosmos only through *prana* at this particular moment. The slightest tension in any part of the body or a minor diversion in attention needs energy and this energy is provided by *prana*. Thus, in order to increase the time for *kumbhaka*, it is important that all other requirements of the body are suspended. Each part of your body should be in rhythm with the intake of the vital energy.

In *kapalabhati pranayama*, you are supposed to push out the air from your lungs. This process should involve only your respiratory mechanism, the rest of your body should be completely still. Check your arms, legs, shoulders and every other part of your body to make sure that they are in a completely relaxed state. Think of a sleeping baby whose body is completely limp and relaxed and try to copy this, not with sleep but with a conscious effort. You will realize that when you are successful in staying completely relaxed during *pranayama*, you will slowly be able to increase your capacity to prolong *puraka*, *rechaka* and *kumbhaka*.

EIGHTH WEEK

A. *Pashchimottanasana* or the Forward Stretching Posture

This is an important asana for those who have a curve in their thoracic vertebrae and have a posture defect due to their shoulders bent forwards. There are various reasons for this defect. Some people have bent shoulders because they have had them like that from their childhood and nobody ever corrected them. Some women told me that they began to bend their shoulders at puberty because they were shy of their breasts. Many desk workers also have this defect. They work in a slightly wrong posture and over the years the curve in their shoulders increases. This defect may not be troublesome in youthful years but at a later age (40 onwards), it may give rise to pain in the arms, shoulders and thoracic region of the back. Thus, it is advisable to work on this defect while there is still time to cure yourself with this asana.

This asana is done in three steps (Figs. 59-61). Lie down straight on your back, completely relax and slowly stretch your arms upwards (Fig. 59). Those who have forward-bent shoulders will not be able to hold their arms straight in this posture. Their arms will be curved and will be lifted from the floor. Such people may limit themselves to only this part of the asana for the time being along with the regular practice of 6 backbone asanas. They should gradually try to attain this posture with straight arms. If you have already spent thirty years of your life with bent shoulders, do not

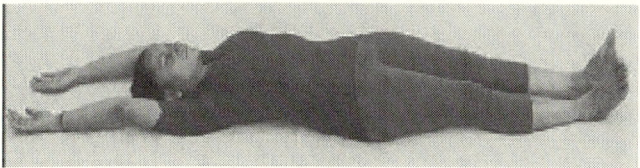

Figure 59 *Pashchimottanasana*

expect to cure it in a few weeks. If you have perseverance, patience and a strong will to cure yourself, you will certainly be successful. It is also very important to be conscious of this defect in order to correct oneself continuously to get the shoulders straight. Sleeping on a hard bed is equally essential.

The next step of this asana is to slowly raise yourself from the waist without moving your legs and with your head parallel to your arms (Fig. 60). Bend forwards very slowly in a smooth motion until your hands can touch your feet. Hold your feet with your hands and stay in the asana as long as you can comfortably (Fig. 61). You will feel that your back muscles and the lower muscles of your thighs and calves are stretched. Your abdominal and thoracic muscles will be contracted and so will the internal organs of these regions. While in this asana, concentrate on the form of your body in this posture and check that you are free from the tension of the effort you made in order to attain this posture. Recover from the posture by taking off your hands from your feet and slowly straightening your back. Breathing is automatically regulated during this asana. When you begin to raise yourself from the horizontal position, you will inhale, while bending down, the air is partly pushed out and at the time of recovery, the rest of the air is also exhaled out. If you sit longer than a few seconds in this asana, breathing continues slowly. Repeat 5 to 10 times and gradually increase the time of the asana.

Possible difficulties: One principal difficulty relating to the first part of the asana has already been discussed. The second major difficulty faced by a large number of persons in the West is that they simply cannot get up without the support of their elbows. When they try to raise themselves from position one, they are unable to do so and instead their

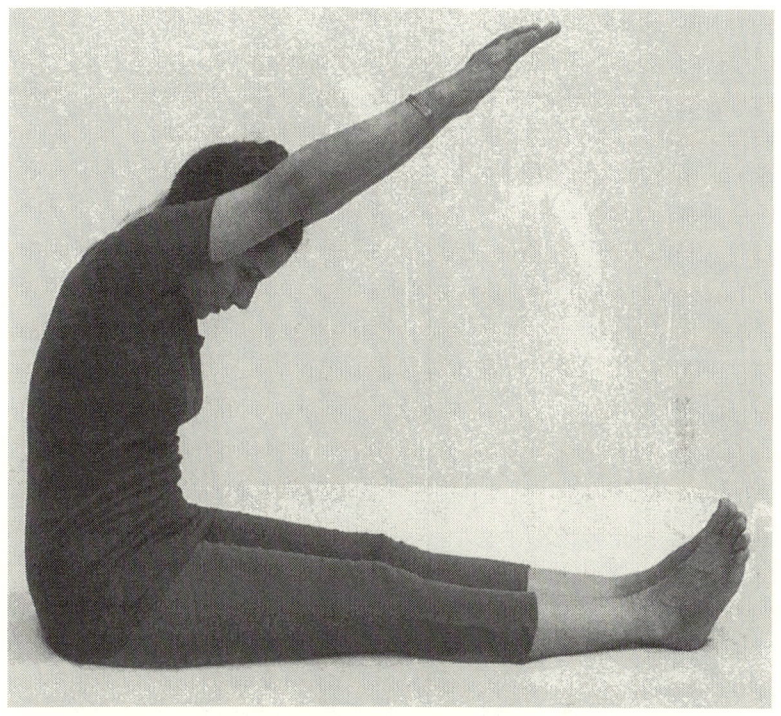

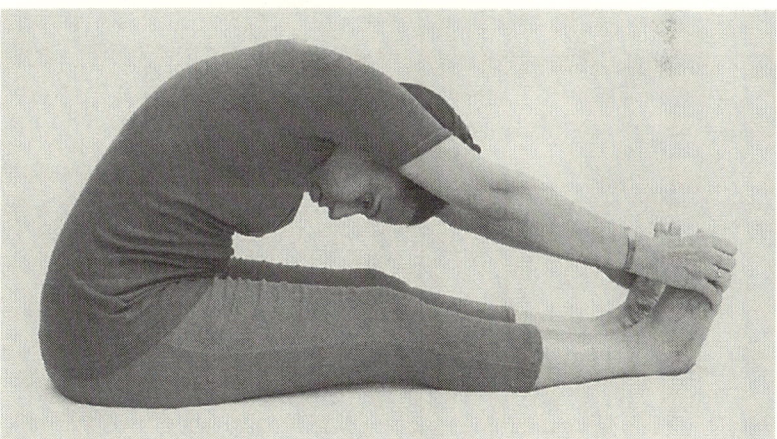

Figures 60 and 61, *Pashchimouttanasana*

legs lift up. The reason for this is that they try to get the force to get up from the upper part of the back instead of from the lower part. It is possible that due to a lack of proper exercise, their lower back muscles are weak. If you have this problem, let somebody hold your legs gently to the ground when you try to get up from the horizontal position. This way, you will get a feeling for applying force on the right part of your back in order to get up without the support of your elbows. The lower back muscles will slowly get stronger in this process.

Benefits: This asana is good for the whole body and brings vigour to the face. It strengthens the spinal cord and makes the vertebral column flexible and elastic. It is a very good asana to ensure the proper functioning of the kidneys, liver, spleen and large intestines. It is recommended to those suffering from haemorrhoids.

B. *Hasya Yogabhyasa* or the Laughing Yogic Practices

The name of this *yogabhyasa* might sound funny to you but the principle is the same here as for the other yogic practices, i.e., to develop an ability to control one's actions, movements and other activities. Here are two different practices that teach you how to attain consciousness about the process of laughing. These practices will make you realize how many different parts of your body are used in the simple act of laughing.

1. Sit down in a comfortable position. Begin to laugh loudly with your mouth open. Gradually laugh louder and louder, and as fully as you can. Continue laughing without restraint for about a minute or until you can stop. In my yoga classes, I mostly had to wait about 10 minutes before everybody could stop laughing.

2. This practice is unlike the above as you are supposed to laugh with your mouth shut and without moving your facial muscles. You should laugh internally and there should not even be a smile on your face. Your eyes will become bright during this practice and you will feel that each part of your body is laughing.

Possible difficulties: Some people cannot laugh loudly. They are inhibited and restrain themselves. They have difficulty in expressing themselves fully. They should try their best to develop the ability to do this *yogabhyasa*. It will do them tremendous good and help them to get rid of their inhibitions in general.

Benefits: During loud laughing, you will realize that abdominal muscles are greatly involved in this process and it provides exercise to the lungs and the lower part of the throat. Laughing without restraint helps to get rid of inhibition and releases tension. Quiet laughing teaches self-control and demonstrates how in the process of laughing your whole body participates.

C. The Subtle Body—*Nadis*, *Chakras* and *Kundalini*

We have already talked about the subtle body within the human body (see Chapter 1, and Week IV, E). Now we will discuss this subject in more detail in order to understand the basic concept of yogic powers and the distribution of energy in the body.

I repeat again that the subtle body within the human body is not to be confused with the anatomical systems of our physical body. The word *sukshma* or subtle denotes on the one hand the invisibility and on the other hand the superiority over the physical body. When we say that "*prana* invades our whole body or we can guide *prana* to a particular part of our body", it refers to our subtle body within our body. The ancient Indians knew that the air we breathe in goes to our lungs, as they had explored the anatomy and physiology of the body. The subtle body represents the whole cosmos within us. We are a part of this cosmos and in elemental form we are the same as the rest. The cosmos is made up of five elements—ether, air, fire, water and earth. This elemental power is distributed throughout our body as follows: 1) earth is between the feet and the knees; 2) water is between the knees and the anus; 3) between the anus and the plexus is light; 4) between the plexus and the eyebrows is air; and 5) between the eyebrows and the top of the head is ether. In Tantric literature, these elements are represented by different symbols with different colours. In the present context, I will not go into the details of these symbols. The interested reader may refer to other books on the subject (see Chapter 1, reference 14).

In addition to the five elements, the subtle body is made up of a network of channels or *nadis* through which circulation of *prana* is made possible. We have already discussed the three principal *nadis* in the programme of the IV Week. *Sushumna nadi* is straight and is in the middle of the back whereas *ida* and *pingala* cross *sushumna* and each other at six different points. The final meeting point of the three *nadis* is at the level of the anus where *kundalini* or the dormant psychic power lies. The meeting points of the three *nadis* represent the confluent points of energy and are called *chakras*. The corresponding points of *chakras* are shown in Fig. 62. Only *sushumna nadi* goes beyond the forehead, up to the top of the head where the seventh chakra is located.

When the adept of yoga has achieved mastery in *pranayama* and is able to isolate him or herself from the external world, then he or she is able to perceive the subtle body.

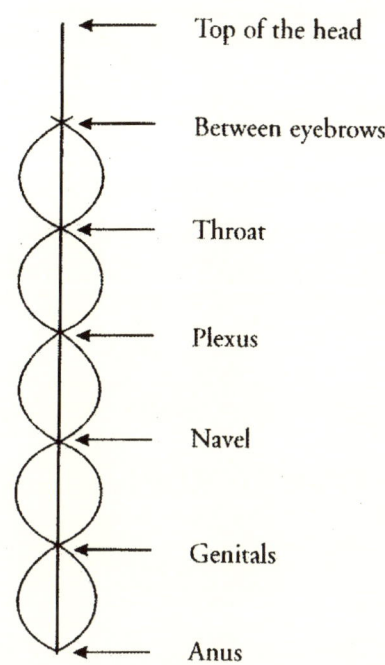

Top of the head

Between eyebrows

Throat

Plexus

Navel

Genitals

Anus

Figure 62: *A diagrammatic representation of the three principal channels of the subtle body and their intersection corresponding to six chakras.*

The *kundalini shakti* is in the form of coiled energy lying at the base of the three major *nadis*. It is dormant in the normal human state and thus is coiled up. It is also referred to as serpent power because it is figuratively represented by a coiled serpent. The task of the adept is to awaken this dormant power within him or herself. In other words, to awaken the *kundalini* means to achieve conscious awareness of the presence of the cosmic power within us.

It has already been said that the individual soul is a part of the Universal Soul and that this latter is the essence of all existence (see chapter 1). The subtle body represents the energy provided by that essence and *kundalini* in the subtle

125

body represents the dormant and unused source of that energy. To put all this in very simple words, we can say that there are three steps of the ladder: 1) our physical being; 2) the subtle body which represents the cosmic energy within the gross body (physical body); and 3) the soul which is the essence and the animating principle of all beings. The soul is the cause of subtle body and the subtle body is the cause of physical body. In this brief description of the subtle body, it is not possible to go into details of *chakras* and their figurative forms etc. Table 2 shows the names of the *chakras*, their corresponding *mantras*, vital activity and their function.

Table 2. The seven energy chakras, their mantras, vital activities and functions

Chakra	Symbolic sound or mantra	Vital activity	Function
Muladhara	*Lam*	Sense of smell	Governs lower limbs
Svadhishthana	*Vam*	Sense of taste	Governs arms and hands
Manipura	*Ram*	Sense of sight	Governs excretion
Anahata	*Yam*	Sense of touch	Governs sexual organs
Vishuddha	*Ham*	Sense of hearing	Governs oral activity
Agya	*OM*	Mind	Governs all forms of mental activity
Sahasrara	It is beyond all, it denotes Brahman	Denotes the termination of the journey of Kundalini	

When the *kundalini* is awakened by the power of *pranayama, pranava japa* (recitation of "OM") and other yogic practices, it ascends through these *chakras* awakening their latent energies. These *chakras* are the source of *siddhis* or occult powers the adept attains through the practice of yoga (for details of various *siddhis*, see Patanjali's Yoga Sutras, Part III). In fact, the rise of *kundalini* denotes various stages of consciousness an adept undergoes before reaching the final goal of yoga, i.e., to free the soul from the cycle of birth and death (*sansara*) and unite it with the Universal Soul. The journey of the *kundalini* ends at *sahasrara chakra* which is located on top of the head, and signifies its reabsorption into *atman* (*Purusha*). This is the state of *kaivalya* or the total isolation described by Patanjali. The individual soul is separated from the Universal Soul only as far as it is involved with the Cosmic Substance—*Prakriti*. Once the soul is separated from the Cosmic Substance, it unites with the Universal Soul and the adept is liberated from *sansara*.

This is an extremely brief description of the subtle body. I feel, nevertheless, that it will help you to know the basic concepts essential in understanding various yogic techniques and their application.

In the present context, it is important to learn well the practice of *pranayama* and to develop an ability to guide *prana* into the desired parts of the body. This is achieved through long-term practice of *pranayama* and *ekagrata* or single pointedness of the mind. The energy for pursuing any goal, whether it is for maintaining good health or attaining a *siddhi* or healing oneself, comes from within us. Our energy remains unused because of a lack of knowledge and effort. It is exclusively through our own efforts that we can awaken the body's dormant energy. It is only by the consciousness of this energy within us that we can connect ourselves to the Universal Energy and be in harmony with it.

Do not think that only some people can evoke the dormant powers and can attain *siddhis*. Although outwardly, we may all look different, we all have a similar elemental form, a similar subtle body, similar soul and thus, similar capacities. According to the Yoga philosophy, the external and situational differences between human beings are due to their accumulated *karma* (previous action) and *sanskara* (accumulated impressions of the previous actions). Human freedom lies in the ability to use the infinite capacities within us.

D. *Dharana*, *Dhyana* and *Samadhi*

Patanjali puts beautifully the purpose of *pranayama:* *"Tatah, kshiyate, prakashavaranam"*, i.e., "That, (practice of *pranayama*) weakens the obstruction of light." (Part II, sutra 52). It means that the light is within us but it is obstructed by *avidya* or ignorance. We get involved in this world and begin to think that we will remain here forever. We seek happiness in this world from others, from objects, from material goods; forgetting that all this, including our physical self is as temporary as a bubble of water. When the "obstruction of light is weakened", we are able to recognize the light within us and realize that the happiness is within us. We are able to know our true self which is beyond our mortal self. For this realization, we need a thought-free mind. It is only by the power of the mind that a continuous flow of thoughts in the mind is controlled. If the human body is compared to a chariot, the mind is a set of reins (see Chapter 1, quotation 13). The word 'body' is used here to designate our whole physical being along with our mind and intelligence (*buddhi*). It is the mind which directs the chariot to reach its destination. Through the preceding pages of this book, you have been learning to give this training to your mind so that it develops the ability to control itself. It is only through very small steps that one can learn this.

'Meditation', 'consciousness', 'being conscious' or 'universal consciousness' are much talked about words these days. An effort is being made by so many organizations and groups to bring awareness about these subjects. In spite of that, it seems that the profoundness and the essence of these words have not been fully understood. One cannot aim at achieving collective consciousness, universal consciousness and cosmic consciousness until one begins with the awareness of one's own micro-cosmos—the human body.

The word 'meditation' is very loosely used in the West these days. Many young people follow gurus from the East who give them a 'secret word'. They sit down and repeat this word without knowing its significance and call this 'meditation'. In technical yogic language, this kind of repetition of a *mantra* is called *japa*. It is done to harmonize the mind and to bring it to concentration. There are two currents of thought flowing in the mind. When you are doing *japa* (this is what we did by the recitation of "OM"), a background current of thought may also be there. To get rid of this current of thought, we try to engage our mind on the figurative form of "OM". The idea is to completely concentrate on the Universal Power and to forget entirely the phenomenal world. This is a first step towards meditation. There are other stages of consciousness between *japa* and meditation or *samadhi*. This latter is a state of cosmic consciousness where identity of the self is lost.

In Table 1, I have summarized eight yogic practices described by Patanjali. The last three yogic practices are: *dharana*, *dhyana* and *samadhi*. *Dharana* is the next step after *japa*. It is the concentration of the thinking principle (*chitta*) on a single point. This point does not belong to the external space as the senses are completely withdrawn during *dharana*. Thus, in *japa*, there is a repetitive sound whereas in *dharana,* concentration is limited to the internal space—*desha*. It means that one concentrates on the subtle points of energy in the body, the chakras, which we have already talked about in the preceding pages.

When the state of *dharana* is maintained continuously, this is called *dhyana*. *Dharana* can be visualized as continuous drops of falling water whereas *dhyana* is like the flow of a liquid with a thick consistency like oil.

Patanjali defines *samadhi* as follows: "*Samadhi* is when (*dhyana* reaches a state where) only awareness of its meaning remains and (even) the personal identity is lost." (Part III, sutra 3).

It is well known that the sages went to the forests to be alone in order to attain a state of meditation. *Rishis* or seers were able to become one with the Universal Soul and could leave their bodies for months and years. Examples of such sages who live in the uninhabited areas of high Himalayan Mountains are still found. All this is to stress that a state of *samadhi* or meditation is not something which is attained in a meditation centre, with a group and in the hearts of large metropolises. In this book, we will confine ourselves to the correct usage of terms according to the technical language of yoga and will advance further on this path taking into consideration our limitations. If we are able to spare some time to work on ourselves in order to control our thought process and to obtain some peace with *japa* and *dharana*, this, in my opinion, is already a great achievement. If we set very high aims for ourselves and do not realize our limitations, we may end up with no progress.

NINTH WEEK

A. *Sarvangasana* or the Whole-Body Posture

As the name suggests, this asana involves the whole of our body and provides exercise to all organs. Lie down on your

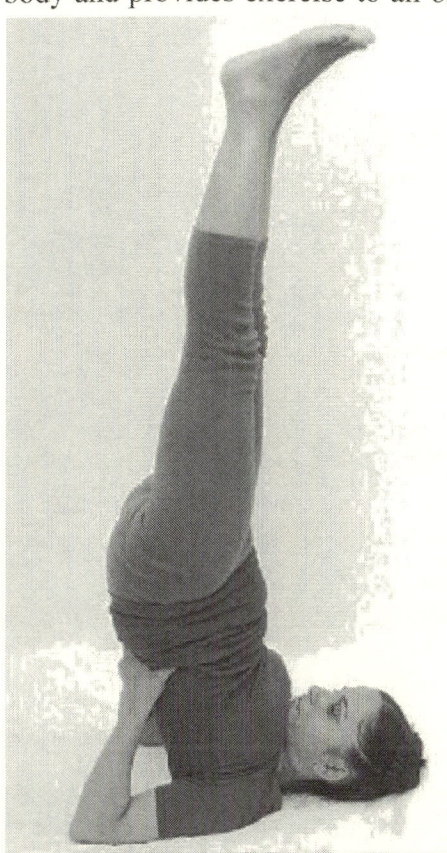

back with both hands at your sides and legs together. Slowly raise your legs as you did for the raised-leg posture (see Week I, C, Fig. 16). When your legs are at a right angle to your body, stay for a few seconds like this and then slowly bring your legs towards your head. Your waist will be slightly raised in this process. Now slowly put your hands on your back to provide a support. Then

Figure 63 *Sarvangasana*

straighten your legs and with the support of your hands straighten your whole body. Your head, shoulders and your hind arms (arms from shoulder to elbow) should be touching the floor, the rest of the body should be pointing straight up in the air (Fig. 63). Your chin will be pressing against your chest in this asana. Breathing will be slowed down as the air cannot enter very deep into the lungs. Stay in this asana as long as you can comfortably. To recover from this asana, slowly bend your legs forwards (towards your head), remove your hands from your back and gradually let your back descend to the floor. Bring down your legs slowly to touch the floor lightly. Do not make this asana or recover from it with a jerk. In the beginning, stay in this asana only for a few seconds and gradually increase the time up to 3 minutes. After this asana, relax in *shavasana* for a while.

Possible difficulties: It takes time until one acquires an erect posture. The thoracic region supports most of the body weight and one feels a great pressure in this region during this asana. The chin presses into the chest, the internal organs are hanging upside down and one may feel some pressure in the chest.

Benefits: We spend most of our time in a vertical position and there is an enhanced blood flow towards our feet. This asana does a great deal of good to the body by increasing the blood flow in the opposite direction towards our neck and head. It is helpful in treating disorders of thyroid, tonsils, neck lymph nodes, ear-nose-throat passages and sinus. It strengthens the nervous system and is good for eyesight. It brings a glow to the face. This asana is very good for a general well being of the body.

Caution: Those who have any problems with their cervical vertebrae or have an injury in the shoulder region should not attempt to do this asana as well as the following two asanas.

B. *Halasana* or the Plough Posture

As the name suggests, this asana consists of making the shape of a plough with your body. Lie down on your back with your arms at a little distance from your body and legs together. Relax completely. Slowly raise your legs as you did for the previous asana. Move your legs towards your head. Stay a few seconds like this. Advance your legs further towards your head by raising your back until your feet touch the ground beyond your head (Fig. 64). Your knees should not bend and your arms and hands should not move in the process of making this asana. As in the previous asana, the breathing is automatically regulated. Since the air cannot enter very deep into the lungs while in this asana, breathing remains very superficial. Stay for a few seconds in the beginning and gradually, with practice you may learn to stay in this asana for up to 3 minutes. Recover slowly from this posture by slightly raising your legs first and then by touching the floor with your back. Now gradually lower your legs from the right angle position and softly touch the floor. Relax in *shavasana* after this asana.

Optional: When you feel comfortable in this asana and can stay for up to one minute in this position, you may place your arms upwards like in figure 59 and touch your feet with your hands.

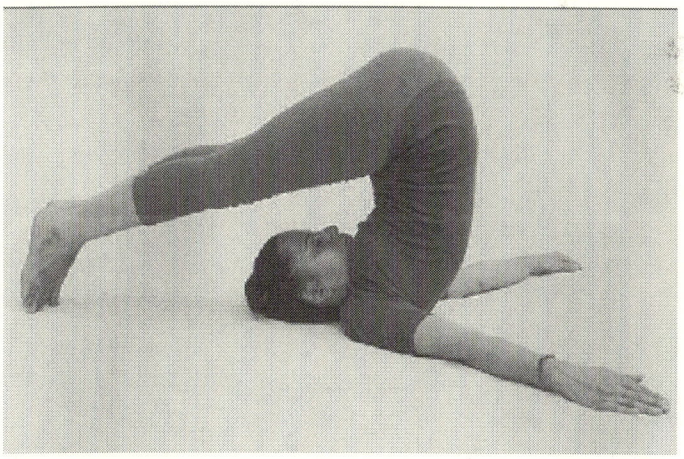

Figure 64 *Halasana*

Possible difficulties: Some people may not be able to move their legs far enough back in order to touch the floor with their feet. This is due to a lack of flexibility in the back.

This flexibility can be gradually attained with practice. Move your legs as far back as you can each time. You will realize that slowly your waist will bend more and you will be able to achieve your goal.

Benefits: This asana is useful in making the body supple internally as well as externally. It is good for the digestive and excretory systems. Like the *sarvangasana*, this asana also enhances the blood flow in the head and neck regions. It also helps keep a youthful vigour and is good for slimming.

C. *Ushtrasana* or the Camel Posture

Sit on your heels in such a way that your knees are about 30 cm apart. Then slowly straighten up until you are "standing" on your knees. Put your hands on your waist. Gradually bend your back from your waist and neck. Bring your hands to your back and put the palms of your hands on the soles of your feet (Fig. 65). Stay in this asana as long as you can comfortably. Slow breathing will continue during this posture. Recover from this position by putting back your hands on your waist, straightening up again and finally to sit on your heels. Relax in this position (*vajrasana*, second version) for a while. With gradual practice, increase the ability to stay in this asana longer.

Possible difficulties: Some people may feel dizzy in this asana. If this is the case, do not stay in this posture. Return to the starting position immediately and repeat several times. Do not do this asana when you are tired. It may cause dizziness.

Benefits: This asana distributes the body's energy, brings equilibrium of *gunas* and thus, insures good health. It corrects digestive disorders, increases blood flow in the head region and makes the body supple.

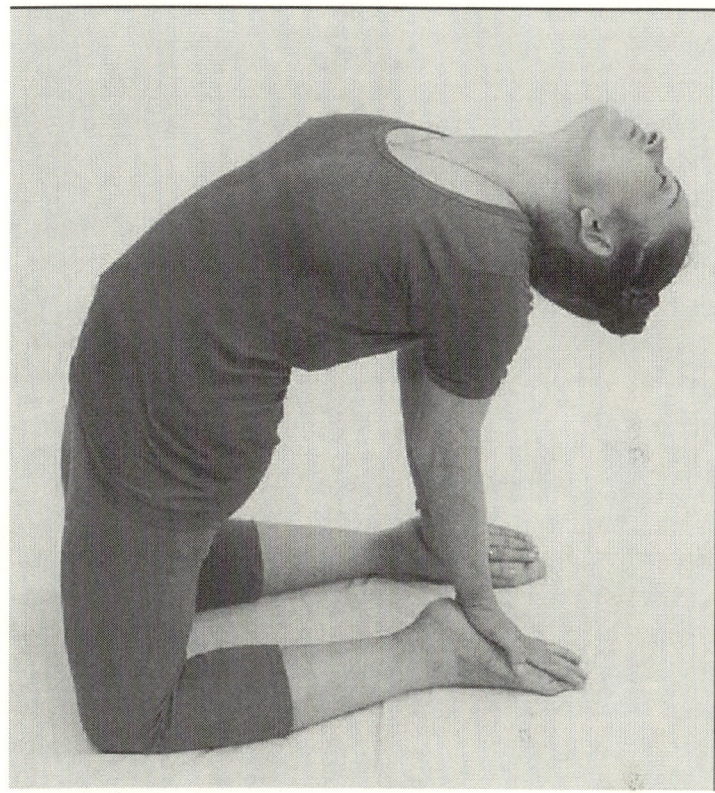

Figure 65 *Ushtrasana*

D. Initiation into *Dharana*

In last week's program, I mostly described the theoretical aspects of mental concentration. Here are the various steps in attaining *dharana* and the techniques for each step.

During the course of this book, various techniques are taught to keep the mind from wandering. Total attention is brought to the body by concentrating on yogasanas and other yogic practices to obtain a *single pointedness* of the mind or *ekagrata*. The *japa* of "OM" has also been done to obtain a thought-free mind. It is time now to revert back to the subject and discuss various aspects of it relating to individual variations before taking the next step of the ladder.

Some of you may find that it is easy to concentrate on yogic practices whereas it is very hard to obtain a thought-free mind otherwise. As I said in the beginning (see Chapter 2), achieving a thought-free mental state is fundamentally a matter of training. To achieve a stillness of the mind, one has to train oneself to develop an ability to control one's mind. This is not done only by holding a daily half an hour session but also by constantly developing an ability to bend one's mind. I come back again to my favourite example of language learning. Learning a new language for half an hour daily will certainly help but what really brings about advancement is your repetitive effort to speak the language. Some people learn a foreign language in school for 6-7 years but are unable to speak as compared to others who learn it only for a few months in the native country and are able to speak reasonably well. It is by training and repetitive force that the mind acquires knowledge of any new system, be it a language or the concentration practices. During a language-learning process, you give your mind directives to assimilate new words, sentences, grammatical forms, etc. For obtaining a thought-free mind, you have to give directives to your mind to detach from the external world and reach a state of stillness. You are trying to stop ripples (the thought process) in disturbed water (the mind) in order to see a clear image of the moon (soul, the true self) in the water.

In the preceding text, I have described various methods for training the mind in order to achieve stillness. But you may follow alternative methods or you may invent your own methods. You may choose any sound or word or music or a visual form that pleases you. Repetition of two lines from your favourite poem done with a perfect concentration will also help stop the ripples in the mind. I do not recommend looking at a flame or your finger while moving it closer to your eyes. Such practices are injurious to the eyes. It is better to close your eyes and imagine the form you want to concentrate on rather than staring at an object.

The major benefit of *ekagrata* that one can put in words is the experience of calmness and stillness. The experience of inner joy obtained from *ekagrata* cannot be explained as it is a very personal experience for each one of you. Those of you who have the conviction and courage will go in for this experience.

The initiation into *dharana* is done with the pre-supposition that you have background knowledge and you have been regularly practicing the yogic asanas, *pranayama*, *japa* and *ekagrata*. All these practices form a foundation for initiation into *dharana*. During the practice of *dharana*, the senses are closed from the outside world. The mind concentrates on the elemental form of the body or one of the *chakras*. For practising *dharana*, choose a quiet and airy place. Sit comfortably with folded legs on a cushion or a carpet. Do not face a source of light. If it is night time, switch off the lights or if it is daytime, draw the curtains or face away from the window. This is done in an effort to shut yourself off from the external world in order to see the internal light.

Begin the session with *pranayama*, and then do recitation of "OM" by visualising its figurative form. Gradually drop the sound and merge in completely with the inner music of "OM" and its figurative form. With closed eyes visualize the figure of "OM" in the middle of the two eyebrows at the place of *agya, chakra*. "OM" is the mantra for agya chakra. At this time, the only reality which should exist for you is this mantra; there is nothing else in the world.

It is easier said than done. All sorts of thoughts try to penetrate the mind. In yoga texts, it is said that the mind is

137

attracted to the world as a magnet to iron. The thoughts slide into our mind even without our wanting them. You will have to learn to seal your mind and to keep the thoughts out. Your attention will be diverted again and again and you will have to make an effort to bring it to the form of "OM" again. This will keep happening. Do not get discouraged; be patient and remain firm on your path. You should do this practice every day. The best time for it is either before going to bed at night after cleaning your mouth and washing your hands and face or early in the morning after evacuation and a shower or a bath. For more details of concentration practices with mantra OM, please refer to my book, *AUM: The Eternal Energy*.

The practice of *dharana* will enable you to see your mind. It will measure the degree of tension and stress you have in your mind of which you may or may not be aware of otherwise. The inner disturbances make the ripples stronger in your mind and you will find it more difficult to bring it to stillness. This practice will enable you to see, the accumulated dust on your mind and persistence in it will enable you to clean this dust. A poem in Hindi comparing the mind to a mirror says the following:

**"Your mind is like a mirror, it sees all,
it sees all; good and bad both.
One cannot hide anything from the mind, it has thousands of eyes.
Oh Creature! Don't let the dust accumulate on this beautiful reflecting glass."**

Chapter 4
Health Protection, Healing and Menstrual Problems

The Western world's way of reacting to bodily ailments and malfunctions is very different to ours. Aches and pains are probably the most common of human complaints. When somebody complains of a headache in your family, the quick response to this in the West is to extend your sympathy to the suffering person by offering a pain reliever. I grew up in a family where three generations lived in the same house. If somebody complained of a headache, the others offered this person a head massage and a cup of tea. It was also common to be given a head massage before examination from one of your family members. The interfamilial massage is a kind of healing massage which is mostly done by pressing as you learnt in the first yogic practice of this book (see Figs. 4, 5). There were also professional massage men and women who came to the family from time to time to give a stronger oil massage. Besides massage therapy, the other frequent remedy for ailments in Indian homes is the nutrition therapy. In Indian cuisine, a large variety of spices, herbs and other condiments are used which not only make gourmet meals but also provide an apothecary. This knowledge is the wealth of familial traditions and is unfortunately getting lost amongst the urban population.

The hectic life in the cities does not leave enough time for people to take care of each other and to cure each other by releasing the stress through pressing and massaging and by redistribution of the body's energy. People have little patience for herbal cures as they find them very slow reacting. They find the painkillers too convenient. Thus, in the evolution of our civilization, the consumption of industrial chemicals is on the rise. Nutrition therapy along with the specific use of various seeds and herbs are extensively described in my other books (see the booklist at the back).

Every minor pain is a kind of a warning from our body and it should be attended to and followed by cure and rest. These days, when people have a headache, they continue their work or entertainment after saturating themselves with painkillers. The frequent and long-term use of such drugs gives rise to stomach and/or kidney problems. The most frequently used and the most well known pain-relieving drug that is in a large number of commercial pain-killing medicines is acetyl salicylic acid. An excessive use of this drug has not only been found to cause a lack of appetite and give stomach ulcers but also decreases the blood clotting factor in the body. Thus, it increases the menstrual blood flow and can cause a serious problem in case of an injury. This discussion is in no way to condemn the drugs and the modem medical system in general. It is to control an excessive consumption of industrial chemicals which may be damaging to our system. Alternative methods of using natural medicines and mild medicines accompanied by healing practices are sought in order to minimize the intake of strong industrial drugs into our body. In this direction, our first effort should be towards maintaining good health, rather than being negligent, falling seriously ill and then being in need of strong drugs.

Health Protection

The origin of a large number of our ailments is to be found in emotional problems. They are an expression of our accumulated emotional stress. We know that nothing gets lost in nature. There is a constant change and conversion and all the elements are recycled. Once we pollute our atmosphere in one way or the other, there is nothing we can do about it. We have to suffer the consequences either in terms of our health or our vegetation on this globe. A few years ago, we did not know that the release of certain substances from our industries would cause ozone depletion in the atmosphere. Ozone is a form of oxygen which is present in the atmosphere (about 20 to 45 kms above the ground) and prevents the sun's ultraviolet radiations from coming to the earth. The ultraviolet radiations are damaging and cause skin cancer. I am narrating all this to underline the fact that all incidents, all aspects of our living and all our experiences leave a permanent mark on us. They may not be in our conscious memory, but they are there. They leave their mark in one form or the other on our existence. The accumulative negative experiences express themselves in the form of ailments. All of us have different weak points where expressions of stress appear. Some of us get stomach ulcers, others get migraines; some get pain in their left (or right) shoulder while others have their sensitive point in the pelvic region. The question is what to do about it. As long as we live, we cannot completely avoid negative experiences, sorrow, pain and stress. But nevertheless, we can learn to change our point of view and can work on ourselves so that we do not accumulate the effect of sorrow, pain, stress etc. Learn to deal with the problems there and then. Do not push them aside and do not stack them. Reason them out and learn to see your own mistakes rather than always sympathizing with and pitying yourself. Learn to look at others with compassion and learn to forgive. This is not to be done for the sake of others but for yourself and for your peace. Do not live in an unhappy situation for too long. Do something to get out of it. Do not feel helpless. There is always a new way in life. The accumulative effect of day-to-day unhappiness is disastrous and ruins health.

Save yourself from stress as much as you can. Remember that stress is a mental state and it is in our hands to get rid of it. You are late, the bus does not come on time, there is a traffic jam and you are helpless. In such a situation, even wrecking your nerves will not help you to gain time. Then why not save the nerves at least; the time is lost in any case. There are thousands of such situations in our daily life. We should consciously work on ourselves and train our minds to stay calm even in the worst of circumstances.

About 40 years ago, when I was still a little girl, cancer was a very rare disease in my country. Nobody knew this word 'cancer'. I had heard my grandmother talk about an incurable boil. She said that this was a sign of accumulated worries and grief which expresses itself in the form of a deadly boil. There is a proverb in Hindi which says "Worry is like a funeral pyre". Scientists may feel proud to cause stress to the poor rats in their laboratories to prove what all stress can produce but the fact is that this wisdom has been known to human beings from time immemorial.

The second aspect of the health preservation is physiological. It is to activate your body's defence system (immune system) and to prepare yourself against a possible future attack. For example, if people around you have some sort of infection of the throat, larynx, etc., you may become vulnerable to this infection. You should use a bi-directional preventive method against this attack. The first step consists in fighting against the attack physically, i.e., taking preventive measures like gargling, throat cleaning *yogabhyasa*, drinking large quantities of liquids, specially hot water with lemon and other teas to this effect. The second step consists in doing *pranayama* practices and concentrating with *prana shakti* on the vulnerable or affected part. Tell yourself again and again that you are not going to get this infection and that you have the power to defend yourself against this attack. Not tiring yourself excessively, taking regular meals and getting enough sleep are some other factors that you should pay attention to.

Healing

Healing is not something mysterious as it is sometimes viewed in the West. It involves bringing oneself to a complete restful state and then directing one's energy to the ailing part. The *single pointedness* of the mind or *ekagrata* is focused on the ailing or recovering part of the body. With the power of the mind, one vitalizes the suffering part by redistributing the body's energy.

The part of the body to be healed should be personified. It will bring a distance between this part and your thoughts. Then you are able to talk to this part of your body. Concentrate on the affected part and converse with it in a very tender and affectionate way. Tell this part of your body to have courage, to show bravery and be healthy. Pat it softly and then tell it that you will provide it, with extra energy to get healthy. Do *pranayama* practices and guide the *prana* to this part. Hold the *prana* there and concentrate on the affected part to nourish it with positive energy and take out its negative energy. When this exchange is done, exhale the negative energy completely. Repeat this process several times. For this process of healing, an appropriate condition of rest and comfort should be created for the organism.

There are times when pain or the malfunctioning of an organism or mental confusion is too much and you feel that you have no energy and initiative for self-healing. At such times, you require another person to heal you. For healing others, you need to establish a connection with the other person and with his/her ailing part. Put your hand on the affected area of the other person and through this, transfer your *prana shakti*. Do the rest in the same way as for self-healing.

143

Your ability to heal and degree of healing depends on your power of concentration and mastery in *pranayama*. The more your mind gets trained in *single pointedness*, the more you get the power to heal.

For chronic pains, one should carefully study the symptoms before the disorder expresses itself. If you are attentive, you cannot miss the pre-warnings of frequent pains. One can work on the problem at an early stage and can attain success in warding off the disorder. There are always some circumstances which trigger off chronic pains. We have to cure ourselves by removing the causes and creating a suitable environment for making the weak part healthy.

Menstrual Problem[18]

In the context of health protection, it is important to discuss about menstrual problems from which half the humanity seems to suffer in one way or the other. Headaches, restlessness, depression, abdominal pains, indigestion are the frequently heard complaints caused by hormone changes. A regular practice of asanas (specifically those where it is indicated) cures this problem to quite an extent. But for a complete remedy and a feeling of well-being, women should also pay attention to other things:

- Always eat a large amount of vegetables and fruits and avoid fatty foods.
- Make it a habit to drink water in the mornings. Problems of constipation should be completely eradicated.
- Drink a lot of fluids, especially 15 days before your menstruation.

---

[18] *For more details of Women's ailments, see my book: The Kamasutra for Women. This book has also been translated into German, French, Portuguese, Dutch, Italian, Hindi and Malayalam*

- Soak 8 to 10 almonds in water the night before and eat them the next morning after peeling off their skin. Do this every morning for 15 days before menstruation.

There is practically no cure in modern medicine for the problems caused by menstruation except giving additional hormones. Some people think that since medical sciences have been almost exclusively in the hands of men until recently, there are very crude and primitive ways to cure health problems concerning women. However, in traditional cultures, women themselves held these domains and there are various simple methods to provide relief from menstrual troubles. In India, there is a well-known cure provided by professional massage women: the abdominal massage. There are several other Ayurvedic recipes with simple and easily available products generally used as spices (see my book *Kamasutra for Women*).

Chapter 5
Summary and Conclusion

Progressive Learning

Those of you who already know about the yogic practices and its philosophy may find this book very unusual because the most classical and well-known asanas like the *padmasana* or lotus posture and the asanas of *suryapranama* or salutation to the sun are not mentioned here. I wish to offer something from which people can learn and understand and which can help them to make yoga a way of life. According to my practical experience, more than 99 percent of the people in the West or urban people in general have physical difficulties which prevent them from making complicated asanas. Besides, people do not have relaxed mental states. They are hyperactive and when they are told to relax, they often become more tense. I did not want to make this book formidable by beginning with something which most of you find difficult to deal with. More important than learning to make a particular posture is to acquire a calm mental state and develop the ability to control one's mind. This process takes time and requires your total attention. It is harmful to give one's body physical shocks by forcing oneself to twist and turn in certain ways. Thus, I propagate a very gradual way of learning. For more complicated asanas, consult my various books on Ayurveda as well as *Patanjali and Ayurvedic Yoga*.

You need not follow the prescribed number or time duration for yogic practices and yogasanas. I have stated them to give you an approximate idea. It is better that you develop your own feeling for time according to your capacity.

I have described some very fundamental and basic practices which are very important and which are often not mentioned presuming that they are very personal and that people know them already. I have designed this book to provide a good foundation which will lead you to do a solid construction for self realization.

Teaching Yogic Practices to Children

You can teach children some yogic practices with the help of this book. Here are some instructions to this effect. You may start teaching your child at the age of two and a half or three years. At this age, the yogic practices have to be taught in a playful manner by trying to show the child the imitations of the postures of animals the asanas are named after. It is only after the age of 6 years that they begin to understand the importance of concentration as at this age they are trained to concentrate at school. Children will do the movements very fast. You should not interrupt them and let them do the way they like. Later, you can tell them through an indirect suggestion that how wonderful it feels to do the same thing slowly. The advantage of teaching yogic practices to children at such a young age is that their bodies continue to be flexible and they develop the capacity to stay in an asana for a long time. If you continue to teach them, they will gradually begin to understand the discipline in its entirety. In fact, children should be taught about the value of concentration by indirect suggestion rather than direct imposition.

Comprehension

Another aspect which is extremely important is a complete comprehension of the subject and its aim before you decide to take up this path. You should understand it, approve of it and then follow it with conviction. The path of yoga should not be taken because others do it and it is a fashion. Doing anything without understanding well can be very dangerous.

In this context, I am reminded of an incident. When I was living in Washington, I had a friend who often complained that her boy friend went regularly to some meditation centre in the city and that he mystified various aspects of their relationship because of this. One day she came to me in a rather desperate state and asked me, being an Indian, if I knew what flying meditation was. I really did not know what to say to her as it did not make any sense to me. My ignorance on the subject made her all the more desperate and she announced her decision to leave him because he was doing some kind of flying meditation but could not explain to her what it was. She was convinced that the man she was living with was slowly going mad and decided to leave him before he completely lost his head. I pitied that young man who not only let himself be misguided by some guru but also lost his girl friend.

The subject of yoga should not be treated differently from any other kind of learning. It should not be considered as something mysterious. There are many questions and doubts in the West about the *siddhis* (unfortunately translated as miraculous powers). As much as the Western nations are advanced in the anatomical, physiological and molecular aspects of the brain, as backward are they in knowing about the capacities of the mind which *rishis* (seers) of the East had explored thousands of years ago. The Western scientists want to prove the power of the mind in the laboratory. They fall in a trap in this process. The mind has to be expanded to use its full power. The instruments which are developed by an "unexpanded mind" are limited and cannot prove the power of an expanded mind.

Self-Help for Health

During my numerous discussions with various people around the world on the subject of self-help for good health, I found that there was a category of people who admitted their total incapability to do something for themselves in

149

this direction. These are not the people who were sceptical about my ideas on health but were the ones who basically would have liked to do something for themselves in this direction but felt incapable. They find it hard to stay alone, quiet and without doing anything. The movements of the yogic practices are too slow for them and their mind's attention span is not long enough for that.

This problem is understandable. It is the mind which controls mind. Somebody with a weak power of mind finds himself/herself incapable of proceeding with this process. Actually, the situation is not so hopeless for the weak-willed and nervous persons. It is only made hopeless by their fear. One must work on oneself and prepare oneself by telling oneself again and again—"It is possible, I can do it, I want to do it." Think about the many other things in life which you can do and do well. Be encouraging and kind to yourself. Think that to obtain a state of mental concentration, you require a similar effort as for doing other things. If you can cook a good meal, paint a wall, grow plants, repair broken cars, put tiles on a leaky roof or hundreds of other such activities, then how can it be possible that you cannot develop a capacity to bend your mind. You need mental preparation for getting self-confidence and this latter will give you a capability to help yourself with your own power of mind.

Belief

Some of you might have this misconception that by doing yogic practices or *japa* you are stepping into some beliefs which are not yours. On this subject, I would like to add two points. I will say my first point in the words of Alain Danielou:

"The word 'Hindu', used for convenience, can be misleading, for it may convey the idea that Hinduism belongs to a country, to a particular human group, to a particular time. Hinduism, according to the Hindu

150

tradition and belief, is the remnant of a universal store of knowledge which, at one time, was accessible to the whole of mankind."[19]

Secondly, I feel that old traditions and cultures do not belong to an exclusive group, they are our heritage as universal citizens. There are people of different races, colours, nations, beliefs on this earth but we are all bound to each other by natural forces. We live on the same planet, it is the same sun which provides energy to all of us and makes life possible on our planet. We have the same moon and the same stars. Our gods may be different, the shapes of our places of worship may be different but we cannot deny our basic unity through universal energy.

Yoga and Women

There is a misconception that yogic practices are exclusively for men and that the feminine word for yogi 'yogini', means witch or female demon.[20] I cannot explain how this word 'yogini' came to mean that, however, I can speculate on the subject by taking examples from the living traditions of India. It is a well-known historical as well as actual fact that some people use their *siddhis* not for the purpose of yoga (i.e., to attain oneness with the Absolute) but for their selfish motives like destroying their enemies or doing something else in this direction. There are many instances in recent history (especially from East India) that women misused their yogic powers to take revenge for their suppression by the family. This was especially true in case of the widows who had to lead a very restricted life in some sections of the society. Possibly, this was the beginning of this interpretation of the word 'yogini'.

---

[19] *Alain Danielou, The Gods of India: Hindu Polytheism, page X, 1985, Inner Tradition International, New York*
[20] *Jean Varenne,* Yoga and the Hindu Tradition, *page 65, 1976, The University of Chicago Press, Chicago*

The meaning of the word 'yogini' is not of much significance to conclude the exclusivity of yoga for men as in the living tradition, the women who work for their liberation from sansara are addressed as *ma* or mother. There are many women like that all over the country, living in temples or exclusive huts at holy places. Both men and women pay homage to them.

Yogic practices and asanas are done by both men and women equally. I learnt yogasanas from my father. My mother never showed any interest in such activities. At my school, which was a girls high school, yogasanas were taught in the extracurricular activities. The path of yoga is in no way closed for women.

As for the negative comments on women concerning yoga in some ancient texts, I would like to say the following. Indian culture is very ancient and is extremely rich in philosophy and literature. It has flourished on a land which has always known freedom of thought. There was always somebody in the past, as is also true for the present, who did not feel quite at ease with the opposite sex. Indian culture is exclusive in the world in doing research on the equilibrium in male and female energies and feminine energy is considered as a power or *Shakti*.

Yoga and Society

In this book, I have discussed various things which we can do for our health. However, "doing for ourselves" and "caring for ourselves" should not make us self-centred and over occupied with ourselves. The self awareness should make us more tolerant and generous towards our fellow beings. Taking care of oneself should not be confused with pampering oneself. Patanjali says, "The mind is purified by friendship, compassion, tenderness equally towards happy and unhappy, kind and unkind humans" (Part I, sutra 33). If we wish to take the path of yoga, we need to incorporate these qualities in us. This is what we have in our hands and from here we can begin the process of consciousness. Collective consciousness in a society begins with individual consciousness. Most of us are aware that there are other major factors which are hazardous to our health and changing them requires collective consciousness of our societies and ultimately the universal consciousness. We need to save our environment from pollution, we need to stop consuming pesticides with our food, we need to save ourselves from radioactive disasters, we need to stop the consumption of industrial drugs and other such abuses.

I feel that by individual consciousness, we can do very much for ourselves but we cannot do all to ensure good health. However, this is the only way which will unite us in a collective effort to change something on our globe and to work together towards goodwill and good health.

OM SHANTI

About the Author

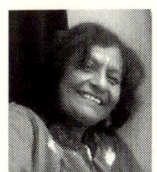 Along with a doctorate degree in reproduction biology in India, Dr. Verma studied Neurobiology in Paris University and obtained a second doctorate. She pursued advanced research at the National Institutes of Health, Bethesda (USA) and the Max-Planck Institute in Freiburg, Germany. At the peak of her career in medical research in a pharmaceutical company in Germany, she realised that the modern approach to health care is basically fragmented and non-holistic. Besides, we are directing all our efforts and resources to cure disease rather than maintaining health. In response, Dr. Verma founded The New Way Health Organisation (NOW) in 1986 to spread the message of holistic living, preventive methods for health care and to promote the use of mild medicine and various self-help therapeutic measures.

Dr. Verma grew up with a strong familial tradition of Ayurveda with a grandmother who had enormous Ayurvedic wisdom and was a gifted healer. She has studied Ayurveda in the traditional Guru-shishya style with Acharya Priya Vrat Sharma of the Benares Hindu University for 23 years.

Dr. Verma is an ardent researcher and is working hard to compile the living tradition of Ayurveda and spread it in the world through her books and other activities. She has published twenty three books on yoga, Ayurveda, Women and Companionship. The books are published in various languages of the world. Besides, she has published numerous scientific articles. Several other books are in preparation. She lectures extensively, teaches in Europe for several months a year, trains students at her two centres in India and gives radio and television programmes. A film on Ayurveda with her was made by German television in 1995 and was shown in 100 countries, in 130 languages. It was the first film on Ayurveda.

Dr. Verma has founded Charaka School of Ayurveda to train interested people with genuine Ayurvedic education so that they can further impart the knowledge of Ayurvedic way of life and save people from becoming a victim of charlatanry in Ayurveda. She is doing several research projects on medicinal plants and their combination in the form of remedies. She is the founder and chairperson of *The Ayurveda Health Organisation*, which is a charitable trust for distributing and promoting Ayurvedic remedies and yoga therapy in rural areas of India. She does regular lectures and workshops for school children in the rural and remote areas of the Himalayas to promote wisdom of traditional science and medicine. Dr. Verma gives seminars, lectures and teaches in the *Charaka School of Ayurveda* with guru-shishya tradition.

For more information and contacts for Dr. Verma's school and teaching programme see www.ayurvedavv.com and www.drvinodverma.com

Dr. Vinod Verma's Publications

1. *Patanjali's Yoga Sutra: A Scientific Exposition* (Published in English, Hindi and German).

2. *Ayurveda for Inner Harmony: Nutrition, Sexual Energy and Healing* (Published in English, German, Italian, French, Romanian and Hindi).

3. *Ayurveda a Way of Life* (Published in English, German, Italian, French, Spanish, Czech, Greek, Portuguese, Slovenian and Hindi).

4. *The Kamasutra for Women* (Published in English [America and India], German, French, Dutch, Romanian, Italian, Portuguese, Slovenian Hindi and Malayalam).

5. *Stress-free Work with Yoga and Ayurveda* (Published in German, English [America and India] and Hindi).

6. *Patanjali and Ayurvedic Yoga* (Published in English, German and Hindi).

7. *Programming Your Life with Ayurveda* (Published in German, French, English, Slovenian and Czech).

8. *Ayurvedic Food Culture and Recipes* (Published in English, German, Czech and Hindi).

9. *Yoga: A Natural Way of Being* (Published in English, German, French, Italian and Hindi).

10. *Companionship and Sexuality: Based on Ayurveda and the Hindu tradition* (Published in English and German).

11. *Natural Glamour: The Ayurveda Beauty Book* (Published in German, Spanish and English)

12. *Losing and Maintaining Weight with Ayurveda and Yoga* (Published in English, Slovenian and German).

13. *The Timeless Wisdom of Ayurveda: A Scientific Exposition* (Published in English and German)

14. *Prakriti and Pulse: The Two Mysteries of Ayurveda* (Published in German)

15. *Good Food for Dogs: Vegetarian nourishment based on Ayurvedic wisdom* (Published in German and English)

16. *Diet for Losing Weight* (published in German and English)

17. *Aum: The Eternal Energy* (Published in German and English)

18. *Pulse Diagnose in Chinese and Ayurvedic Medicine* (co-author for TCM Dr. Florian Ploberger) (published in German)

19. *Shiva's Secrets for Health and Longevity* (published in German and English)

20. *Healing Hands: The Ayurvedic Massage workbook* (published in English)

21. *Prevention of Dementia* (published in German and English)

22. *Ayurveda for Dogs* (published in German and English)

23. Numerology: Based on the Vedic Tradition (published in English and Slovenian)

The Charaka School of Ayurveda and Patanjali Yogadarshana Society (Himalayan Centre)

The Charka School of Ayurveda (CSA) has been founded by Dr. Vinod Verma to spread the genuine classical tradition as well as the living tradition of Ayurveda in the world for promoting healthy living and preventing ailments. Its aim is to teach people a healthy lifestyle which enhances immunity and vitality and enables them to live a life with an optimum level of energy. For minor ailments, people should be capable of using home remedies, appropriate physical and mental exercises and nutrition.

CSA aims to bring genuine and practical aspects of Ayurveda to people and save them from Americanised and Europeanised distorted versions of Ayurveda and other forms of charlatanry that do more harm than good.

To achieve this purpose, CSA organises to train students in Europe who can further spread the message of Ayurvedic lifestyle and help people with genuine massages, purification practices, nutrition and other practical aspects of Ayurveda. The school is in association with the most learned persons of Ayurveda in India and several exclusive persons involved in health education in Europe.

The object of Patanjali Yogadarshana Society is to spread the message of Patanjali in the world. The wisdom of the Yoga Sutras is not only beneficial for the yogis but also for our day-to-day normal life. Its aim is to enhance *sattva* or the inner stillness and peace in the world as well as in the individual minds. With years of research on Yoga and Ayurveda, Dr. Verma has founded the Ayurvedic Yoga and has written a book on the subject.

Lectures, Seminars and Training Programmes

To get detailed information on the Charaka School of Ayurveda as well as our other programmes in India and Europe, visit our website or contact us by email.

The New Way Health Organisation .NOW.

A-130, Sector 26, Noida 201301, U.P., India

Tel. 0091 (0)120 2527820 or (0) 9873704205 or (0)9412224820
www.ayurvedavv.com www.drvinodverma.com
Contact at: ayurvedavv@yahoo.com

Himalayan Centre

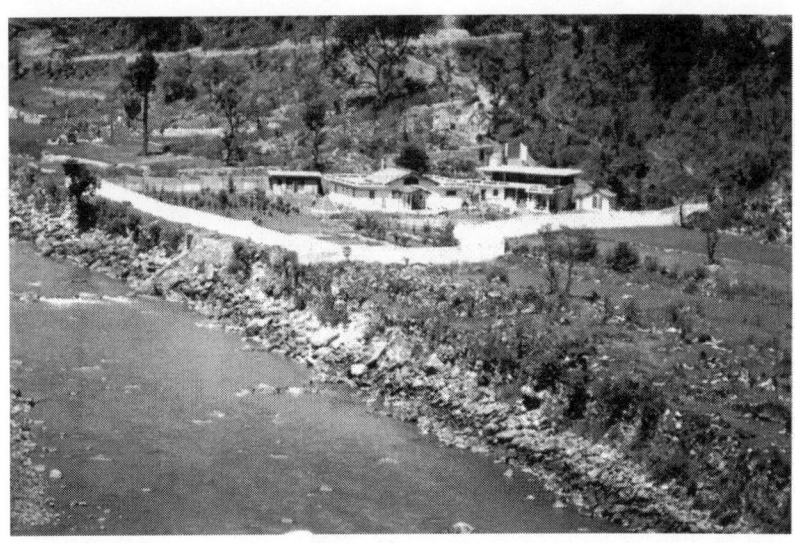

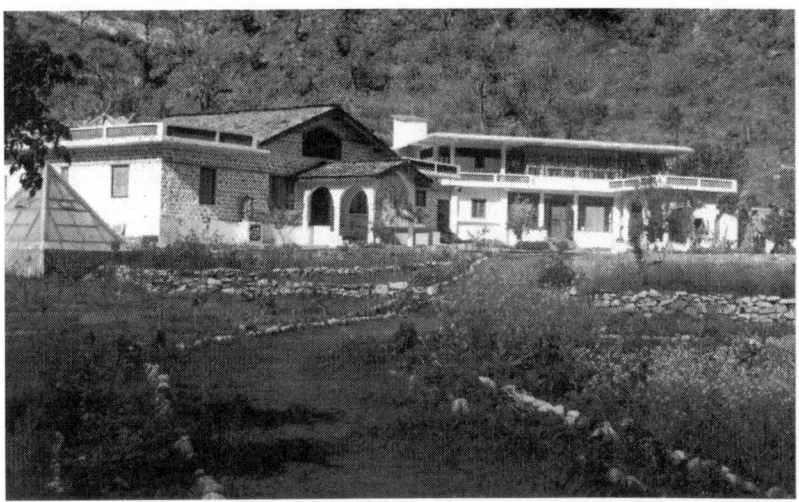

Companionship and Sexuality in Ayurveda and the Hindu Tradition

This book is not available in the market any more. We have some limited edition in four colours and can be directly

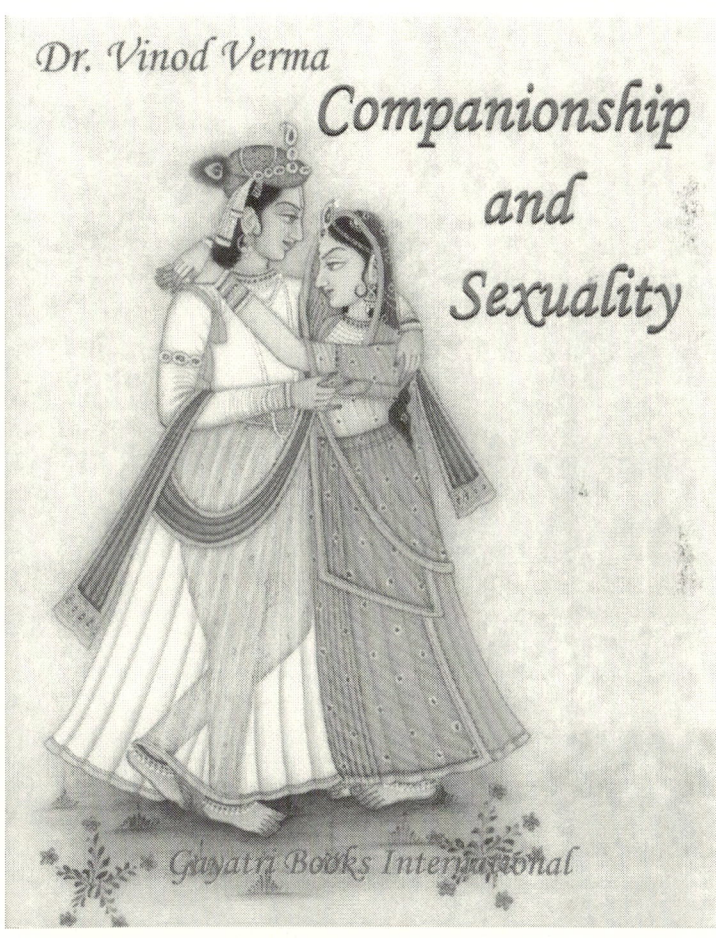

ordered with us. The book costs 39 $. For a special price, (29 $ including postage) please write to Vanaja Vishal at ayurvedavv@gmail.com..

Here is a little description about the book.

Companionship and Sexuality

Sexuality is considered holy in the Hindu tradition and intense sexual experience leads to the cosmic bliss. One of the eight disciplines of medicine in Ayurveda is devoted to sexuality and rejuvenation. Sexuality is also considered as the basis of existence in terms of cosmic continuity in Ayurveda, as well as in other scriptures of the Hindu tradition. Based on this tradition, the author has analysed the primordial differences between men and women due to the different ratio of the three characteristic qualities of the Cosmic Substance— sattva (stillness), *rajas* (action) and *tamas* (inertia). Both men and women should make efforts to understand each other better by accepting these differences, as well as taking into consideration the individual variations due to the fundamental constitution (*prakriti*) described in Ayurveda.

It is suggested that the education in companionship and sexuality should be imparted in an organised way to young people just as it was done in ancient India by the Ganikas (a special group of women who imparted this education). The book provides analysis and practical aspects of this education.

We have made a lot of progress in communication at technological level and our globe is like a village now. However at the level of intimacy between man and woman, we apply the ancient norms, which are not holistic and are based merely on need and convenience. The book emphasizes that in the modern times we need to change the way we look at a man-woman relationship. Just as we would not like to wear the clothes people wore a century ago, similarly, we should not use the old and redundant way of looking at a man-woman relationship as need-based alone.

Rituals and ceremonies are given to intensify the companionship and enhance sexual energy. There is a description of numerous aphrodisiacs to solve specific problems that hinder the flow of sexual energy and to enhance the sexual compatibility.

79748176R10098

Made in the USA
Columbia, SC
29 October 2017